ENVIRONMENTAL BIODYNAMICS

Environmental Biodynamics

A New Science of How the Environment Interacts with Human Health

Manish Arora
Paul Curtin

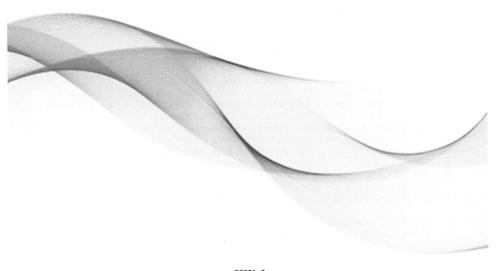

With
Austen Curtin
Christine Austin
Alessandro Giuliani

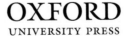
UNIVERSITY PRESS

OXFORD
UNIVERSITY PRESS

Oxford University Press is a department of the University of Oxford. It furthers
the University's objective of excellence in research, scholarship, and education
by publishing worldwide. Oxford is a registered trade mark of Oxford University
Press in the UK and certain other countries.

Published in the United States of America by Oxford University Press
198 Madison Avenue, New York, NY 10016, United States of America.

Library of Congress Cataloging-in-Publication Data
Names: Arora, Manish (Manish Kumar) author. | Curtin, Paul (Paul C. P.), author. |
Curtin, Austen, author. | Austin, Christine (Christine Enid), author. |
Giuliani, Alessandro, 1959– author.
Title: Environmental biodynamics : a new science of how the environment
interacts with human health / Manish Arora, Paul Curtin ; with Austen
Curtin, Christine Austin, Alessandro Giuliani.
Description: New York, NY : Oxford University Press, [2022] |
Includes bibliographical references and index.
Identifiers: LCCN 2021031355 (print) | LCCN 2021031356 (ebook) |
ISBN 9780197582947 (hardback) | ISBN 9780197582961 (epub) |
ISBN 9780197582978 (ebook)
Subjects: MESH: Environmental Medicine—methods |
Precision Medicine—methods | Environmental Exposure—adverse effects |
Environmental Pollutants—adverse effects | Time Factors
Classification: LCC RA566 (print) | LCC RA566 (ebook) | NLM WA 30.5 | DDC 613/.1—dc23
LC record available at https://lccn.loc.gov/2021031355
LC ebook record available at https://lccn.loc.gov/2021031356

DOI: 10.1093/oso/9780197582947.001.0001

1 3 5 7 9 8 6 4 2

Printed by Integrated Books International, United States of America

Contents

Foreword

Complex systems cannot interact directly or exist in isolation. With this short and seemingly simple statement, Manish Arora, Paul Curtin, and their colleagues have written a marvelous book for those who are passionate about the environment. They have planted a seed for a bold idea that hopes to bring about an advance in the way we understand our relationship with our environment and how it impacts human health.

From 2009 and 2019, I served as the Director of the National Institute of Environmental Health Sciences (NIEHS), the preeminent governmental funding agency worldwide for environmental health research. During my tenure I provided leadership and management to thousands of government-sponsored research projects that have greatly enriched human knowledge on environmental health, a field that complements genomics in exploring the determinants of health and disease. I often stressed that nothing is just genetics and nothing is just environment, but our health is a combination of both contributing factors.

One inspired project was from a young scientist who had completed an eclectic PhD spanning oral pathology, nuclear physics, and analytical chemistry. He proposed a unique idea—that teeth were akin to our body's "hard drives" or the history of a tree's life is reflected in its growth rings. He believed that by determining chemicals along the growth rings in teeth he could build a "map" of a person's history of exposure to various environmental exposures, including those that happened before birth. That scientist, and dentist, was Manish Arora. From those early days as a postdoctoral trainee, he became the first NIEHS recipient of the National Institutes of Health (NIH) Director's New Innovator grant for environmental health sciences and was awarded a Presidential Early Career Award for Scientists and Engineers (PECASE), the highest honor the United States bestows upon early career scientists and engineers, by President Barack Obama. At that point, I invited Manish to give the plenary lecture before the NIEHS Advisory Council. He emphasized that time must be placed at the core of the gene-by-environment understanding of health; just as Newton's and Einstein's theoretical work propelled physics into new frontiers, environmental health sciences required some fundamentally new approaches to bring about a bold new frontier. Four years later, I was thrilled to see that Manish and his distinguished colleagues have realized that vision and proposed a new theory (the biodynamic interface conjecture) and a novel subfield of environmental health sciences—Environmental Biodynamics.

Having had the pride of guiding Manish in his career from a trainee to a full professor, I was honored when Manish asked me to write the foreword for this book. In the simplest terms, this is a book full of fearless ideas, a book that makes the reader wonder how the universe is so diverse but at the same time organized by essential rules, and most importantly, it asks if there are similar fundamental rules that govern how our environment shapes our lives. This book also argues against the reductionist trends that have crept into medical research that have attempted to study our environment and our physiology by breaking them into ever-smaller constituent parts. Instead, Arora and colleagues propose a new elegant view of examining the choreography of interacting systems by considering the whole rather than just the parts. In a recent editorial, published in the journal *BioEssays*,[1] the theory espoused by Arora and Curtin was described as follows: Although we can describe how a human system, such as the endocrine system, works, and likewise the chemical nature of compounds present in our environment; but the result of the interaction is more than a simple combination of the two knowledge sets: We need to study not only the components of a complex system but also the processes that create the phenomena that we witness as a result of this interaction. This is the "biodynamic interface," and it is a conceptual structure that comes into being upon interaction of the component entities; it is a new way to study interactions in complex systems and better understand emergent phenomena. The authors not only make this theoretical argument but have also provided data on how their ideas can be implemented in practice.

This book is strewn with little gems—there is a puzzle for readers to show how a dynamic system may be mistaken for a static one entirely because of our point of view; a famous painting by Marcel Duchamp reveals how time can be placed at the center of our worldview; a poem that conveys the usefulness of "nothing;" and an example of how the chemicals in our blood, such as cholesterol or zinc, actually move in orbits the same way planets do. The passion and effort of the authors become clear through these vignettes and the various sections that provide historical and philosophical context, but it is also clear that the writers desire to share knowledge and be good teachers as they provide tools throughout the book for other researchers and practitioners.

It is my hope that this book will be read widely by students of environmental health sciences and others generally interested in the environment. This work reflects a passionate effort to refocus our profession's view on the importance of time and complexity, to move away from reductionist perspectives that have entrained past generations to envision environmental inputs through static measurements, and to place environmental sciences at the core of the practice of medicine. And, along with the authors, I share my hope that just as Environmental Biodynamics is a first step to a bold new frontier in environmental sciences, there will be many more.

Linda S. Birnbaum, PhD
Scientist Emeritus and Former Director,
NIEHS and National Toxicology Program
Scholar in Residence, Duke University

Reference

1. Arora, M., Giuliani, A., & Curtin, P. (2020). Biodynamic interfaces are essential for human–environment interactions. *BioEssays* **42**, e2000017, doi:10.1002/bies.202000017.

Preface

We are setting forth a new discipline in science, one that we have named *Environmental Biodynamics*. We have done so to recognize that our focus is on the environment and its relationship with our biology, and the key to understanding this relationship is the constant change (or dynamics) of these complex systems. We have also taken a step that is unusual in environmental health sciences—of proposing a new theory, the biodynamic interface theory.

Our collective desire to write this book arose from a shared acknowledgment that many current practices in environmental health sciences needed to be examined through a critical lens—that it was time to leave behind the comfort of opinion and start afresh by questioning decades of dogma. This book is written in the background of the global COVID-19 pandemic, severe weather events driven by climate change, and an upheaval in our social and political systems. All these events only reinforce the importance of our physical and social environment, and how we, as a species, treat this planet. With this in mind, my colleagues and I have written a book that argues for a new, more daring way to look at our environment and its relationship with human health.

Writing this book has been a privilege. I (Arora) was fortunate to be working with friends and colleagues who, like me, are a collection of "atoms with curiosity" (as Richard Feynman put it). There are many people to thank, but I want to start with the unsung heroes of science—the taxpayers who put their faith in us scientists to move the needle forward on the sum total of human knowledge. None of this work would be possible without the generous support of the custodians of federal research funding—the National Institutes of Health of the United States, and especially the National Institute of Environmental Health Sciences. In particular, I thank Drs. David Balshaw, Kimberly Gray, Gwen Collman, and Linda Birnbaum for being champions of academic science. I also want to thank my department chair, my colleague of 16 years, and my friend, Dr. Robert (Bob) Wright, for always supporting my work. I have had the privilege to work with many brilliant scientists, including Dr. Rosalind Wright at Mount Sinai, Dr. Andrea Baccarelli at Columbia University, and Dr. Erin Haynes at the University of Kentucky. They have been inspirations. To my closest collaborators, Drs. Sven Bölte in Sweden, Shoji Nakayama and Miyuki Iwai in Japan, Martha María (Mara) Tĕllez Rojo in Mexico, Andrea Cassidy-Bushrow at Wayne State University, Tanya Smith at Griffiths University, and Renaud Joannes-Boyau at Southern Cross University, thank you for the camaraderie. I also want to thank Lisa Maroski for the many deep and thoughtful discussions at the beginning of this journey. Lastly, but not least, I thank Jill Gregory, medical illustrator at Mount Sinai, for creating all the beautiful artwork for this book.

1

Introduction to Environmental Biodynamics

Introduction

Every day around the world, at the behest of medical professionals, millions of needles are pushed into human veins, and drops of blood are sucked into tubes that pass through highly skilled hands and the most technologically advanced machines to identify components and characteristics of the blood in the form of test results—a set of numbers that is compared to ranges of "normal" values. Presumably, these digits signify the health of various parts of our body, such as the liver, the kidneys, and so on.

Recently, one of those blood draws was mine (Arora); for my annual physical exam, my doctor ordered a complete blood workup—white and red blood cell counts, cholesterol and glucose levels, and about 30 other values. This workup has become a yearly game for us, like darts, to see if my numbers are on target; that is, within the corresponding normal range. Putting aside for now questions about what makes a value "normal" and how those ranges are established, let's consider what one number on one day at one time represents. It's a snapshot; it captures the state of my blood at one moment of my entire life. And, like snapshots, if lots of other factors (such as background lighting and shutter speed for photographs) aren't also just right, then the snapshot might not be a good likeness of me. Snapshots lack important qualities that are inherent in how we perceive the world; they ignore the moments that came before and after and everything else that happens out of frame.

This visit with my doctor made me think of a musical game my wife plays with my triplet daughters on long road trips. My wife hums a song and our daughters guess the name. If they cannot guess it, their mother hums a longer piece of the song until *enough notes (in the proper order)* allow the melody to

Environmental Biodynamics. Manish Arora and Paul Curtin with Austen Curtin, Christine Austin, and Alessandro Giuliani, Oxford University Press. © Oxford University Press 2022. DOI: 10.1093/oso/9780197582947.003.0001

become obvious. It would make no sense to play this game if my wife only hummed one second of one note of the song. Music only sounds like music because of how its components *change over time* and because of the *dependence* of the notes to come on those that have passed.

We can imagine our bodies as an orchestra of many organs and tissues and their cells, each humming complex rhythms but all working together in harmony, a harmony that has been refined by millions of years of evolution. How would we ever know what the symphony made by this orchestra sounded like if we only did one blood test every year? How could this snapshot capture the dependency of each signal in that moment on all the moments that have passed? What if a signal was playing the right "note" in the moment, but was otherwise out of sync with the rest of the orchestra?

A few years earlier I had taken my infant daughters to the pediatrician, and they underwent what is now standard practice, at least in New York—a blood test for lead, the toxic metal that has been linked to many neurobehavioral problems. Remembering my children's fingers being pricked for a drop of blood made me wonder again about that biological orchestra. With all the different substances in our body—the calcium that makes our bones strong, the zinc that helps with immune function, and the hormones that help us mature—what happens when a bad player, such as lead, joins this chemical orchestra? Does it change the rhythm of the whole ensemble, does it play out of sync by itself and leave the other musicians unperturbed, or does it stop the other chemicals from playing altogether?

From these humble beginnings my colleagues and I began a quest to understand how humans and the environment interact and if there are universal rules underlying those interactions. Can we find evidence of such a symphony, and measure its performance as we do with the "notes" of each individual signal? Is there a central theory, like the theories that explain apples falling or why time slows down when we travel faster, that also governs how human physiology interfaces with the environment?

This four-year journey led me to seek the help of scientists and thinkers from different walks of life who originate from the United States, Australia, Ireland, Italy, and India. Each brings her or his own perspectives to the question: *Is there an underlying theory that explains how humans and our environment interact?* This quest led us down many paths, from biology and environmental sciences to theoretical physics and mathematics, even to linguistics, philosophy, and art. The fruit of our labors is a new field of inquiry, which we call *Environmental Biodynamics*. It offers a novel approach to understanding the connections between our physiology and our world—a first step, but by no means the last, in devising a theoretical framework for understanding the relationship between our environment and us.

In our journey to formulate a new perspective on the interaction between the environment and human health, at times we found ourselves with no prior work to cling to, and so we had to lay down the scientific foundations ourselves and then build upon them. At other times we were fascinated and humbled by the work of others and have indicated where we have followed their paths. These words of Denis Noble resonated with me: "there is, a priori, no privileged level of causation,"[1] as did the propositions in Laurent Nottale's work on scale relativity and fractal space-time—namely, that *there are no privileged levels of scale.*[2] Like our work, they have argued so eloquently against the reductionist approaches that have come to dominate scientific inquiry in medical research and assume that measuring something at smaller and smaller scales is somehow going to provide a better understanding of our physiology.

This problem has only increased with recent advances in genomics, proteomics, metabolomics, and other -omic technologies that have propelled the exploration of biology by providing tens of thousands of measures, but almost always as static snapshots. These often-superficial applications of systems theory have neglected the consideration of the fundamental questions that spurred the genesis of the field, which focused on how life is organized and how it functions. Instead, we have created an "ocean of correlation" with an unrelenting modern emphasis on digging deeper and crunching harder, as if including more -omics data and the brute force of supercomputers would miraculously reveal the secrets of how and where we belong in our world. To this end, I found solace in Alfred North Whitehead's notions of the "myth of substance and the fallacy of misplaced concreteness,"[3] because I no longer felt alone in rejecting the view of human physiology and our environment as a collection of things assembled together. Extending from this rejection of "thingness," I always have found it difficult to accept (and I continue to do so) that the "selfish gene" is the main reason why the world is the way it is or why we are the way we are.

Throughout this book my coauthors and I encourage readers to consult other important texts that will enrich their understanding of the topics we weave together. Furthermore, for us it is not enough simply to propose a new field of inquiry or provide a new theoretical foundation; we also see the need to provide tools for others to operationalize Environmental Biodynamics. For this reason, we provide chapters on how data can be collected on the dynamic nature of our physiology and discuss computational methods to analyze those data.

Finally, we also recognize that the principles underlying this new field are themselves dynamic, and our perspective *must* evolve. Our aim is to identify the key principles that scientists will need to build a platform upon which others will stand to advance a better science, one that inspires new ideas, new questions, and new hypotheses. After all, isn't that the ambition of all scientists—to contribute a verse (as Walt Whitman said)[4] so that in time the next verse can be written? Toward this end, we call our colleagues to action and ask for the establishment of the field of Environmental Biodynamics that places the constant change of our physiology and our environment at its core, at the correct dimensions of space *and time*.

What to Expect from This Book

There are many wonderful works that discuss the benefits of healthy lifestyles, such as eating organic food, avoiding certain chemicals, or spending more time in green outdoor spaces; all of those instructions are valuable products of decades of health research. However, this book takes a different route by asking deeper questions to uncover the universal truths underpinning the most important driver of the health of individual humans and human society—our environment. Think of it like this: Isaac Newton did not help us understand how to farm and harvest apples but why and how apples fall to the earth; similarly, we do not discuss how to live a healthy life but why and how the environment influences human health. In the process, we will formulate and present evidence for a new theory and a new scientific field that arises from that theory.

This book is for those who are passionate about the environment, partake in environmental or biomedical research, and/or teach environmental medicine. As such, it is written at multiple levels of complexity; some parts provide a general introduction that is accessible to all readers, and other sections take a deep dive into theories, laboratory methods, and mathematics that are of more interest to scientists actively engaged in this field. We use boxes throughout the book to provide background supporting information relevant to the topics we discuss. We will indicate where we zoom in to technical details so that readers can choose to skip those sections if they are beyond the scope of their interest. We also promise the reader that when we propose a theoretical advance, we will back that claim with real data. And when there are no data, we will clearly indicate the next steps needed to confirm or disprove our proposition so that other scientists may join us on this journey. Each chapter of the book is meant to stand alone to some degree, which is why there are regular "recaps" of material covered in previous chapters so that the flow of our discussions is not interrupted for the reader.

Aims and Scope of Environmental Biodynamics

In emphasizing the need for a new theoretical perspective to guide thinking in environmental health sciences, we have so far neglected some minor points, including: What theory do we need, exactly? And what aspects of our environment and our health should it address? These topics are naturally the focus of this book, but we will first address the general scope of topics that our approach, Environmental Biodynamics, seeks to address.

First, we intend to shift the fundamental perspective on the *complexity* of environmental-biological interactions from the current dogma, which embraces an ever-widening taxonomy of structural relationships, and instead focus our understanding on *functional* interdependencies. In this view, complexity is not a nuisance that obfuscates or obscures our measures or interpretations; rather, complexity itself is what we seek to measure. And while doing so we place that most important of dimensions—*time*—at the core of how we understand the relationship between the environment and human physiology.

Second, we aim to challenge an assumption that is taken as doctrine by many—that complexity should be analyzed and understood at the level of the population or group. This sort of thinking is pervasive in environmental medicine, and not without reason; but, we argue, the time has come to integrate advances in computational and biochemical sciences to finally actualize the promise of precision medicine by studying complexity at the level of the individual.

Last, we seek to illustrate the role that *constraints* play in the measurement and assessment of biological systems, and while doing so we aim to provide new tools to reorient the scientific gaze. Our ultimate goal is to provide a new perspective to organize our study of environment, health, and medicine; to provide, in other words, a new set of questions to ask.

Box 1.1 Structural and Functional Perspectives

One of our goals is to shift the current paradigms in medicine and related sciences, which are predominantly *structural*, to a combined structural *and functional* perspective. The structural perspective focuses on specific aspects of physiology and views them as "things" (organs, molecules, drugs) and focuses on the "what" and "how much" of the environment influences physiology (e.g., which toxin and how much of it causes specific symptoms or a disease, which drug and how much will help alleviate a specific condition). The functional perspective, on the other hand, attempts to understand our physiology by focusing on the *process* of interdependence; specifically, how do interactions that underlie our physiology develop over different timescales, and how do such changes interact with the ever-changing environment? Extending the music analogy mentioned earlier in this chapter, in an orchestra, as one musician is joined by another musician, they each play differently to accommodate the various dynamic aspects inherent in their instruments (for example, a piccolo cannot play the same notes as an upright bass). This then results in a more complex piece of music. This dynamic process of bidirectional interaction and synchronization continues until a harmonious composition is reached. This body of music is, thus, dependent on both the structure *and the function* of the musical instruments, and the same is true for our physiology.

Complexity and the Need for Precision Environmental Medicine

We need first to understand what is *said*, and what is *meant*, when the word "complexity" enters the conversation of environmental medicine. From a standard epidemiological perspective, complexity is a challenge that emerges when we are trying to solve a research problem. And though we say *a* problem, really it is almost inevitably always *the* problem: Does this thing in the environment—maybe too much of a toxic chemical, or too little of a nutrient—relate to human health? Thousands upon thousands of studies, often very nice studies, have been published to answer this exact question, with the specific aspect of health being studied varied each time—maybe brain development in one study, maybe cancer rates in another—just as the specific environmental factor is likewise varied. Complexity, here, is not at the level of the research question, but rather in all the things that make answering that question difficult. Perhaps the toxic chemical has a greater observable effect in one sex, for example, or perhaps we are only sensitive to that exposure when we are children, or the effects are dependent on the dose of the environmental agent. These sorts of challenges are solved with good study design, which in this context means collecting enough samples to deal with this complexity, planning in advance to measure and account for other relevant factors (some would refer to these as "confounders"), and having a statistical analysis strategy in place to model those variables.

Complexity is therefore intrinsic to environmental medicine, and always has been, but notice that this complexity arises along the journey of a research study and is dealt with *in the solution to a research problem*; it is never, in itself, a tool we use in deciding *what question to ask*. One of the pioneers of information science, Warren Weaver, saw the scope of this problem and sought to clarify the types of problems that science investigates. In his seminal paper of 1948 called "Science and Complexity," he proposed three classes of problems—those characterized by organized simplicity, disorganized complexity, or organized complexity[5]—and outlined how these processes can be leveraged to better understand complexity (Figure 1.1).

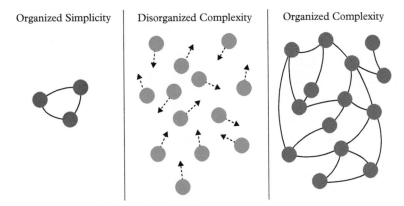

Organized Simplicity | Disorganized Complexity | Organized Complexity

Figure 1.1 Warren Weaver's three classes of complexity. In an *organized simplicity* assumption, a change in one system can be fully explained by a change in another system. Biological systems rarely behave in this manner; inevitably, the number of factors involved, and the complexity of their interactions, precludes such direct exchanges. The *disorganized complexity* scenario assumes a probability-based construct that works on group averages. For example, it provides the average behavior of a group of patients but cannot explain adequately how the environment impacts a particular patient. *Organized complexity* is where this explanation can be found. By focusing on time-dependent patterns we can unravel the bidirectional interaction between systems and operationalize interventions at the level of the individual.

The first class, *organized simplicity*, refers to simple, direct relationships between two systems. This commonly emerges when change in one variable is driven directly by change in another; for example, assuming a circuit of constant resistance, a change in electrical current will yield a corresponding change in voltage. A problem in the realm of organized simplicity can be solved with simple classical quantitative methods (such as a linear, nonlinear, or differential equations). The parameters in the preceding example of an electrical circuit could be solved by Ohm's law (current = voltage/resistance), for example. Organized simplicity nonetheless does not imply that the problems are simple, in themselves. Rather, it merely implies that the relationships in a system governed by organized simplicity are simple or can be simplified. Putting a human on the moon was quite complicated, for example, but it falls into this class of problems because we can directly relate the movement of the earth to the movement of the moon and plot a spaceship's course between them. In part this was because, though the earth and moon are themselves complex systems, and are further subject to more complex forces from the wider solar system, their relative motion and direct interaction could be effectively modeled by treating each as a simple point mass in a differential equation. Weaver suggests that prior to 1900, most problems in the physical sciences were addressed in this way, either through the consideration of only a few variables or through the simplification of systems to equivalent processes. In the last century, particularly following the advent of quantum physics and Schrödinger's uncertainty principle, more sophisticated perspectives have emerged in physics and related physical sciences. But biological studies, generally, and environmental medicine, particularly, have been slow to embrace this shift.

Weaver identified a second class of complexity—*disorganized complexity*—in the organization of physical and biological systems. Disorganized complexity emerges in systems that are characterized by simple, direct relationships, as in organized simplicity, but that involve the interaction of many disparate elements. In such cases the methods used to solve problems of organized simplicity break down (or become exponentially difficult) when there are more than a few variables. It would be easy to calculate the trajectories of two billiard balls, for example, but it would be very difficult, even with modern computational capacities, to calculate trajectories for all of them. However, and rather counterintuitively, if you have a thousand billiard balls, the problem becomes easier because you can characterize their behavior in other general ways by statistically analyzing their overall or average behavior. In fact we face this problem on a daily basis both in practical and scientific pursuits; we cannot possibly measure or predict the motion of individual gas molecules, for example, but we can easily characterize the average behavior of a gas molecule through measures of kinetic energy such as the temperature of that volume of gas.

Instead of using classical mathematics, problems of disorganized complexity thus require a more statistical probability-based approach to solve them. Rather than characterize the motion of any given individual, we seek to characterize the *distribution* of the population—by measuring its average, its variability, and its consistency among other group-level parameters. The caveats for this type of problem, however, are that you must have a large number of the same type of thing (a large number of atoms of a gas in an enclosed volume, for example) and their behavior must occur at random (the technical term is *stochastic*). Characterizing the temperature of a given volume is less meaningful, for example, if one group of molecules has more energy than another. Thermodynamics is naturally a good example of this style of reasoning; we can measure emergent qualities of liquids and gases, such as temperature or pressure, without delving into the microscopic details of each molecule. Paradoxically, this approach is more precise the more numerous the "things" being analyzed, though with each addition we have another characteristic that we cannot evaluate directly but rather only estimate at a group level.

The properties of disorganized complexity, as with organized simplicity, are commonly assumed and leveraged in studies of environmental medicine. The assumption of stochastic processes, for example, is one reason epidemiologists value larger sample sizes (studies with more participants). However, this approach is reaching its limits because the urgent need in medicine is not really about the average behavior of a group; rather, it is quite the opposite—in addition to group behavior, we also need to know the individual's exposure to specific environmental factors and how their physiology is responding to those environmental inputs. Weaver gave an appropriate example in his seminal paper of how this approach works—"it makes possible the financial stability of a life insurance company. Although the company can have no knowledge whatsoever concerning the approaching death of any one individual, it has dependable knowledge of the average frequency with which deaths will occur." This is the very problem we are facing in environmental medicine: A reliance solely on epidemiological approaches tells us what is happening in a population on average terms, but when we visit our doctor, we want to know what is happening to us specifically, which is what precision medicine asks of us (see Box 1.2 for a brief description of Precision Medicine).

Box 1.2 A Brief Note on Precision Medicine

Precision medicine argues against a one-size-fits-all approach to the practice of medicine. Rather, it takes into account individual differences in patients' genes, environments, and lifestyles. In this manner, medical decisions, treatments, practices, or products are tailored to specific subgroups of patients based on their genetic, molecular, or cellular profile. The perceived benefits of precision medicine are to more accurately predict which treatments will be most effective and safe, and possibly how to prevent the illness from happening in the first place. Environmental Biodynamics aims to impact the practice of precision medicine by placing temporal dynamics of our environment and our physiology at the center of medical practice.

The third realm of complexity that Weaver proposed—*organized complexity*—characterizes systems that emerge in a sort of "middle kingdom"; these involve more elements and more complex interdependencies than could be summarized through organized simplicity, but there are fewer elements, which interact through nonrandom processes, to be consistent with disorganized complexity. Weaver describes complex organized systems like this: "They are all problems which involve dealing simultaneously with a sizable number of factors *which are interrelated into an organic whole*" [italics added]. Organic wholes tend to grow, develop, and self-organize, yielding hierarchical systems spanning multiple levels of organization. Consequently, the results are highly context-dependent, which gives rise to the information crisis that environmental medicine is now experiencing. Weaver recognized over 60 years ago that this middle kingdom was the 21st century's frontier of basic science.[6] Since then, mathematical techniques have been and continue to be developed to characterize organized complexity (we use them in Chapter 3 onward and describe them in detail in the appendix).

Weaver claimed that when dealing with complex organized systems, the focus of the investigation shifts from detailed analysis of single elements to perceiving the pattern underlying the connections among those elements; in other words, the interrelationships among the components. This approach pinpoints exactly one of the aims of Environmental Biodynamics: Our goal is to shift the focus of environmental medicine to organized complexity rather than organized simplicity, which treats complexity as a nuisance, or disorganized complexity, which ignores dynamic interdependency (see Figure 1.1). And while doing so, we extend Weaver's work by placing *time* at the core of our approach to studying environment–human interactions.

Contrasting Environmental Biodynamics and Other -Omic Sciences

We are sure the readers have had had their doctor tell them how high (or low) their body mass index (BMI) or their blood cholesterol levels are in relation to a range of normal values (and the same would be true for many other parameters). Consider this, though: *Have you ever been told the "stability," "complexity," or "entropy" of your BMI or your blood cholesterol?* We believe that is exactly what medical tests *should* be reporting to you (and, in Chapter 3, we will show how it's actually done).

Over the past two decades there has been a rise of the so-called -omic sciences: genomics, metabolomics, proteomics, and many others. While the data we present later in this book are generated on laboratory instruments that are also used by -omic scientists, the interpretation is different. In Figure 1.2 we show how Environmental Biodynamics is, in a manner of speaking,

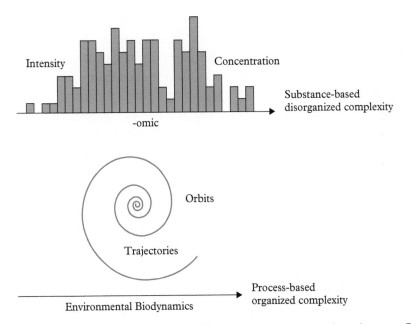

Figure 1.2 Contrasting Environmental Biodynamics with -omic sciences. Current approaches that characterize environmental exposures use measures of concentration and intensity to measure "things" and lead to interpretations embedded in disorganized complexity. Environmental Biodynamics seeks to measure and characterize "processes" to provide an explanation based in organized complexity.

orthogonal to the -omic approaches, and we highlight three key differences. First, the -omic sciences measure many *things*, such as metabolites in the case of metabolomics or proteins in the case of proteomics. Under an ideal scenario, these -omic approaches are embedded in prospective cohort studies so they are measured at several timepoints. In reality, most cohorts undertake measurements every year or two, so if you had a 10-year study, we would have five to 10 samples of blood or urine from each participant on which we could perform our -omic assays. In contrast to this, in Environmental Biodynamics we measure *processes* (not things) in order to understand the organization of trajectories. For example, in one study that we will present in a later chapter, we measured the assimilation of essential and toxic elements at 500 consecutive timepoints.[7]

The second difference between -omic approaches and the methods of Environmental Biodynamics is in the form our measurements take. Under the -omic approaches we measure the "how much" of our targets; for example, the concentration of a metabolite or toxicant in blood. Even when it is a nonchemical target, we measure it in terms of intensity—how intense was the exposure to stress during pregnancy, as another example. However, when trying to analyze Environmental Biodynamics, because we are focused on the nature of processes and complexity, we measure trajectories and orbits—that is, how these process *change* over time—and the synchronization of these processes with respect to other biological variables. The reader will make a connection here with the earlier discussion in Box 1.1 on structural and functional perspectives, and see how the -omic approaches are making a structural interpretation while we are proposing one that is primarily functional (but does not exclude structural components, because they too have value).

The third difference, and perhaps the most profound, is in the final picture that each approach paints. Describing it in terms of Weaver's description of complexity, the -omic technologies lead to a substance-based *disorganized* complexity, whereas Environmental Biodynamics leads to a process-based *organized* complexity. We clarify to the reader that while we do directly compare the two approaches, we are not implying that one is always better than the other or that they are mutually exclusive. Both have value, but at present Environmental Biodynamics is hardly ever used in environmental medicine—and we strongly believe that must change.

Box 1.3 Why Do We Need New Scientific Fields and New Theories?

Fields such as physics and mathematics have many guiding principles and theories that are rigorously debated, modified, and even rejected when evidence emerges. These include famous examples such as the *theory of relativity*. Biology, a foundational science of medicine, also has many theories, the most notable one being the *theory of evolution*. For the most part, environmental health sciences don't work in that manner—data on environmental factors and health measures are collected and we try to uncover the links using statistical methods. If these links are proven to be valid, they can have significant impact on public health. The reduction in exposure to the neurotoxic element lead is one such example of environmental health research success. The improvement in air quality in North America and many parts of Europe is another notable example. With such successes under our belt, one might wonder: *Why ask for the creation of a new field of scientific inquiry?* This is a good question and one we asked ourselves at the beginning of this journey. The reason is that single studies and experiments provide answers to specific questions, whereas a set of principles provides a framework that reaches much further—*it tells us what questions to ask* and connects our answers to a broader framework of scientific inquiry. As a scientific community, we must also recognize that as the component principles and theories of a field are refined, there are many gains that are not always predictable when the field is being developed. Seemingly unrelated observations in our universe become interconnected, sometimes across astonishingly different scales. Further, these principles and theories impart the ability to predict the trajectories of systems and can guide us to correct or modify systems that are headed to an undesirable state, such as the onset of disease. Considering perhaps one of the most recognized theories of all, Isaac Newton was not the first to notice an apple falling to the ground (nor was he the first to propose a theory of gravity; Aristotle and Giovanni Borelli attempted such explanations too). Formulating such observations as a general theory allowed Newton to develop formal equations to quantify the forces of attraction between bodies. Those equations linked the falling apple with the motion of planets and enabled us to launch satellites and spaceships and alter their trajectories when needed. This is not something Newton or his contemporaries could have predicted, and this is why we believe the field of Environmental Biodynamics is needed—so that we can achieve a "moon shot" at a time when we are facing a crisis of our environment in the forms of climate change, unbridled industrial pollution, mass introduction of untested chemicals into our daily lives, and the inability of governments to take timely action.

Principles of Environmental Biodynamics

Complex Systems Cannot Interact Directly or Exist in Isolation

The first and most important principle underlying Environmental Biodynamics, outlined earlier in the chapter, provides the central axiom from which the corollary principles outlined hereafter are developed. This seemingly simple statement, published by us as the biodynamic interface conjecture, is the culmination of many years of work and, as we will show in this book, it has profound implications for how we understand environment–human interactions.[8] Although developed for environmental health sciences, the biodynamic interface conjecture has broader implications for the study of complex system interactions across various levels of organization, the central role of time and temporal dynamics in system-to-system information exchange. This conjecture also argues against causal paradigms that (incorrectly) assume that systems are distinct entities interacting directly and ignore boundary conditions, organizational levels, and complexity inherent in all complex systems. In the remainder of this chapter, we will first unravel the meaning of this conjecture in detail and then we will lay out the corollary principles. The rest of the book is dedicated to showing the impact each principle has on the practice of environmental medicine.

The interaction between human physiology and the environment is key to deciphering the origins of health and disease.[9,10] When examining the health consequences of individual agents or mixtures of environmental factors, studies at all layers of organization, from human populations to controlled experiments on microscopic cells grown in a laboratory, are often conceptualized as a monodirectional causative process with the environment impacting some physiologically relevant, measurable endpoint. In Figure 1.3A, we depict the general formulation of such a research thesis. Examples include the impact of lead exposure on IQ or social stress exposure and levels of cortisol (a steroid hormone) in a biological matrix.[11,12] Positive environmental influences are also conceptualized in this manner; for example, access to green spaces is associated with better measures of cardiovascular function.[13]

While, in practice, many studies adopt this monodirectional approach, all good scientists know that the relationship between the environment and human physiology is bidirectional. Because of this, the arrows visualized in Figure 1.3A should also point from humans to the environment, as shown in

Figure 1.3B. The scenario depicted in Figure 1.3B represents a shift from a simple one-directional perturbation to circular feedback causation within and across levels.[14] A simple example of this is the relationship between human industrial activity and air pollution; our industrial processes increase air pollution and the increased environmental air pollution in turn impacts human health.[15] The nature of this relationship has important consequences in how these systems will evolve over time; in a positive feedback cycle, for instance, increasing exposures will cause more deleterious health effects, which will in turn lead to increased exposures due to greater use of medical facilities that then emit more pollution.

In both panels A and B in Figure 1.3, the often-overlooked aspect is the actual form and physical nature that the interaction between the environment and human physiology can take. Specifically, the underlying assumption is that two complex systems (humans and the environment, for instance) can transfer influence directly to one another. In contrast to this, we conjecture here that *complex systems cannot interact directly*. We propose that the interaction between two or more complex systems requires the formation of an interface (as represented in Figure 1.3C). Further, we contend that the interface is dynamic process–based in nature (Figure 1.3D). This interface incorporates components from all the interacting systems but exhibits *operational independence*. This property has many consequences, the foremost being that the characteristics of the interface cannot be fully resolved by only studying the systems involved in the interaction. The interface must *itself* be the subject of inquiry.

In the principle stated above, of utmost importance is the interpretation of *direct interaction*. From a computational perspective, the direct influence of one system on another implies that the variation in the input/

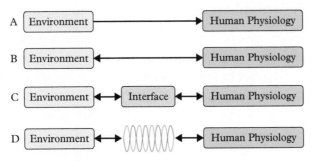

Figure 1.3 Complex systems cannot interact directly but do so via operationally independent biodynamic interfaces.

exposure measure relates to the variance in the output/health measure, even if it is partitioned through other measured characteristics of the systems under study (these are referred to as *covariates* in epidemiological studies). This is the form that many statistical models take when studying the relationship of an environmental exposure on a health outcome and adjust for covariates, and it inherently implies a system of organized simplicity or disorganized complexity. In observational studies, researchers are generally and appropriately cautious in interpreting such associations through the lens of a causal analysis, but the ubiquitous application of this framework nonetheless focuses inquiry at the level of reductionist connections between disparate systems. In contrast, we argue that one or more processes contributing to the interface between systems serves to constrain (or, in more general terms, assign a "meaning" to) what is transmitted to the other interacting system(s). The biodynamic interface, thus, places limits on both *how much of* and *what attributes of* the signals are transferred between interacting systems. This happens in both directions, from environment to human, and from human to environment. The presence and biological relevance of such intermediary processes may be evident in the time-varying dynamics that link environmental and biological systems but may be missed in direct associative studies that seek to link discrete measurements of environmental inputs, often in the form of single measures of concentration, with biological responses.

The axioms we describe next represent the foundational ideas underlying Environmental Biodynamics. These provide an organizing framework around which Environmental Biodynamics can be applied to answer questions about environment–human interactions. The integration of these can provide a new perspective to describe, explain, predict, and most importantly nurture our environment and our health.

Operational Independence

Biodynamic interfaces emerge in the integration of complex systems but are operationally independent of each interacting system. Consequently, the characteristics of an interface cannot be fully resolved by studying the systems (involved in the interaction) in isolation; rather, the interface itself must be the subject of inquiry. Operational independence is not something we dedicate a separate chapter to, but it is interwoven throughout this book as it is essential for each of the other axioms. A general discussion is provided in Box 1.4, but we will explore this topic throughout all chapters of this book.

Box 1.4 Operational Independence

To illustrate in very general terms what we mean by "operational independence," let us start with a hypothetical example that requires no particular medical or environmental science training. This example, we hope, will resonate with everyone from experienced professors sitting in cluttered offices to undergraduate students just taking their first step toward putting their mark on the world of science.

Consider an island in international waters where different countries send their ships to trade their respective products. Country A sends ships laden with goods to trade for other goods produced by Country B. The ships meet at an island in international waters that is at an agreed-upon location. On this island, there are rules that must be followed to allow for equitable trade to occur in an organized manner. Such rules include the manner in which the ships are unloaded and reloaded, an inspection of goods for their quality, an appraisal of their worth so that both sides obtain fair value for their products, and so on. The island functions as the interface by which Countries A and B trade. This interface uses components from both systems (each country's systems involving the production and transport of goods, for example) that are taking part in this interaction. That is, without the ships and products of both countries, the island would have no role to play in trade. But the function of the island is also operationally independent. Knowing the details of the products of each country would *not* allow us to predict *all* the rules that govern trade on the island. However, there is one more important point we must still consider; the physical island itself is not necessary in our example. The trading could in theory occur in international waters at a specific set of coordinates.

This example illustrates an important point about biodynamic interfaces: *They need not be a thing.* The *process* of trading, and implicitly the rules that govern the process (what is allowed and what is prohibited [i.e., the constraints applied by the interface]), is the real interface in this example, not necessarily the physical island.

Scalar Dependency and Relativity

The characteristics of biodynamic interfaces are dependent on the spatiotemporal scale of the observer. Time is at the core of our physiology's evolution, refinement, and function, as well as its interaction with the environment. Therefore, the adequacy of a set of measurements that characterizes the interface guiding a biological system's interaction with the environment is dependent on the temporal resolution of the measurements. A system must be studied at a temporal resolution that is appropriate to the process under investigation. To study population dynamics of a nation, hourly measurements would be inappropriate because it would be too fine a scale of measurement. Similarly, to study the dynamics of a hummingbird's wing flaps, a single momentary measurement in the form of one photograph per hour would be insufficient because the interval between measurements would be too large. Furthermore, the interfaces linking the dynamics of different systems are a function of their dimensionality; that is, they might only be appreciable in certain dimensional states while appearing to be absent in other dimensions. In Chapter 2 we will discuss how our scalar perspective shapes and constrains our analysis and interpretation of biological complexity.

Structured Dynamism: The Shape of Change

Interfaces are process-based and dynamic and exert constraints on the transfer of information between systems. Although the interface is composed of constant change, it retains a quantifiable topography driven by stochastic, deterministic, or chaotic processes. In general terms, the quantifiable topography of an interface includes regular patterns (where a measurable architecture is apparent) interspersed with transitional periods of irregular patterns (where the architecture cannot be discerned). The characterization of these processes—the dynamics of organized complexity—contrasts with the static or a structural perspective of human physiology, which is insensitive to temporal dynamics. Neither regularities nor irregularities can be accommodated in a static or a purely structural view of human physiology. Of relevance to medical practice and research, the concentration of a biomarker of a biological system's performance (a blood test, for example) measured at one or a few discrete timepoints cannot adequately characterize a physiological system. In Chapter 3 we will explore the organization of biodynamic interfaces at multiple levels of complexity.

Dynamic Interdependence

Because complex systems cannot exist in isolation, biodynamic interfaces emerge between integrated systems. These interdependencies facilitate bidirectional interactions between the environment and human physiology. Within our physiology and within the environment, processes do not exist in isolation but are rather interdependent. The temporal dynamics that emerge at one stage of organization reveal interdependencies among proximate processes, which themselves emerge from distal dependencies. In Chapter 4 we will explore how very different stages of biological complexity—for example, the organization of neurocognitive processes, and elemental homeostasis—become connected and interdependent.

Patterns, Forms, and Constraints

The function of biological systems is constrained on multiple levels of organization, and these constraints drive and are likewise driven by the formation of biodynamic interfaces. In embracing the framework of organized complexity, we must recognize that the many dimensions of human health do not simply occur at random but rather are organized according to underlying patterns. Resolving the nature of the biodynamic interface requires an understanding of the bidirectional relationship between the patterns evident in our physiology and the patterns that emerge in functional processes mediating environmental interactions. In Chapter 5 we will explore how the patterns and forms underlying biological systems organize and relate to human health.

Emergent Complexity and Self-Organization

No aspect of the self or the environment is isolated to one level but rather should be studied in the context of self-organization and emergent complexity across multiple levels of biological and environmental organization. In considering the role of an environmental factor we must consider at what physiological level that agent will act, and how dynamics at that level are thereby perturbed. We must likewise explore how these changes propagate to other levels of organization and integrated systems. In Chapter 6 we place Environmental Biodynamics in the context of emergent complexity (an important construct of general systems theory), which drives the formation of novel systems, and how the self-organization of systems yields unique organizational properties at different levels of complexity.

Chapter 1 Summary

To summarize this introductory chapter, we return you to the music analogy we used at the beginning. In order to properly identify and characterize a musical composition, or any dynamic system, it is necessary to identify more than a few isolated "things" making up the pattern. Rather, one must know the sequence of events, and the organization of the system, in order to understand

and recognize the piece. In the same vein, Environmental Biodynamics seeks to understand how the environment and human physiology interact through a focus on functional interfaces; our focus is on the patterns that emerge in our integration of the environment rather than on isolated "snapshots" taken in passing. We highlight the core principle (the biodynamic interface conjecture) and six corollary principles through which this focus can be expanded to develop a new field of scientific inquiry, which we hope will yield new insights into our understanding of human health and disease.

To appreciate the key message of this chapter, select an unfamiliar piece of music, but rather than listen to all of it, skip forward at random intervals and listen to just one second each time. It is unlikely that from these disconnected pieces you will be able to imagine the entire composition. This is very much the problem we are facing in medicine. Our bodies and our environment are constantly changing, and the way they interact with each other is also an everchanging process—we are biodynamic.

Now listen to the entirety of the musical piece you have chosen. If this piece has had any effect on how you feel, you must ask yourself: *How* has this affected me? Specifically, how has this music formed a connection with me? Our proposition is that this piece of music, this complex system that includes several musicians playing in harmony using finely tuned instruments, does not impact you (another complex system) directly. Rather, you put forth a lifetime of experiences and the music meets you halfway to form an interface, which applies constraints to (assigns meaning to) what this music means to you. And this *interface* is the reason why the same piece of music has as many unique meanings as there are people who listen to it. But there is a disconnect between this fact and the way we practice and interpret medical data. If the constant change of our physiology and our environment were like the music you just heard, then we need much more than occasional momentary bits of sound to appreciate the full composition of music. In the same way, occasional blood tests are not adequate to measure our physiology's response to the environment we live in. Environmental Biodynamics is our effort to resolve this problem.

References

1. Noble, D. (2012). A theory of biological relativity: no privileged level of causation. *Interface Focus* 2, 55–64, doi:10.1098/rsfs.2011.0067.
2. Nottale, L. (2010). Scale relativity and fractal space-time: theory and applications. *Foundations of Science* 15, 101–152, doi:10.1007/s10699-010-9170-2.

3. Whitehead, A. N. (1997) [1925]. *Science and the Modern World*. Free Press (Simon & Schuster), p. 52. ISBN 978-0-684-83639-3.
4. Whitman, W. (1892). "O Me! O Life!" In *Leaves of Grass*. https://www.poetryfoundation.org/poems/51568/o-me-o-life
5. Weaver, W. (1948). Science and complexity. *American Scientist* **36**, 536–544.
6. Laughlin, R. B., Pines, D., Schmalian, J., Stojkovic, B. P., & Wolynes, P. (2000). The middle way. *Proceedings of the National Academy of Sciences of the United States of America* **97**, 32–37, doi:10.1073/pnas.97.1.32.
7. Curtin, P., et al. (2020). Dysregulated biodynamics in metabolic attractor systems precede the emergence of amyotrophic lateral sclerosis. *PLoS Computational Biology* **16**, e1007773, doi:10.1371/journal.pcbi.1007773.
8. Arora, M., Giuliani, A., & Curtin, P. (2020). Biodynamic interfaces are essential for human–environment interactions. *Bioessays* **42**, e2000017, doi:10.1002/bies.202000017.
9. Landrigan, P. J., et al. (2018). The Lancet Commission on pollution and health. *Lancet* **391**, 462–512, doi:10.1016/S0140-6736(17)32345-0.
10. Landrigan, P. J., Fuller, R., & Horton, R. (2015). Environmental pollution, health, and development: a Lancet-Global Alliance on Health and Pollution-Icahn School of Medicine at Mount Sinai Commission. *Lancet* **386**, 1429–1431, doi:10.1016/S0140-6736(15)00426-2.
11. Lanphear, B. P., et al. (2005). Low-level environmental lead exposure and children's intellectual function: an international pooled analysis. *Environmental Health Perspectives* **113**, 894–899, doi:10.1289/ehp.7688.
12. Bunea, I. M., Szentagotai-Tatar, A., & Miu, A. C. (2017). Early-life adversity and cortisol response to social stress: a meta-analysis. *Translational Psychiatry* **7**, 1274, doi:10.1038/s41398-017-0032-3.
13. Seo, S., Choi, S., Kim, K., Kim, S. M., & Park, S. M. (2019). Association between urban green space and the risk of cardiovascular disease: a longitudinal study in seven Korean metropolitan areas. *Environment International* **125**, 51–57, doi:10.1016/j.envint.2019.01.038.
14. Noble, R., Tasaki, K., Noble, P. J., & Noble, D. (2019). Biological relativity requires circular causality but not symmetry of causation: so, where, what and when are the boundaries? *Frontiers in Physiology* **10**, 827, doi:10.3389/fphys.2019.00827.
15. Grandjean, P., & Landrigan, P. J. (2006). Developmental neurotoxicity of industrial chemicals. *Lancet* **368**, 2167–2178, doi:10.1016/S0140-6736(06)69665-7.

2

The Lens of "Thingness"

Structuralism, Reductionism, and Simplicity

How Did We Arrive at the Current Worldview of Health?

Our health is so intrinsic to our experience of the world that it inevitably frames how we perceive large aspects of our life. Why are some healthy, and others not; and when, how, and why will one be sick, or healthy again?

And though these questions might be universal, the diversity of answers that have been proposed is staggering in its breadth and scope. From the earliest written records of human existence in Mesopotamia and Egypt we have accounts describing the resilience of the human body, and our efforts to sustain it against the forces hostile to it. These have ranged from the near-cosmic afflictions ascribed to spiritual forces and foes, to the prosaic ails assigned to bad diets and injury, or to shortages in (debatably) life-sustaining alcohol. But whether originating in science or superstition, observation or enlightenment, Bronze Age theology, Greco-Roman philosophy, or Middle Ages ideology, all our questions about human health have inevitably converged on three common paths.

The first of these is in our own nature; that is, the *endogenous* origins of human health. We hear this repeated *ad nauseum* throughout history and find it recapitulated today in genomic sciences. Addressing the origins of human health and disease along this path deals with questions about our inherited qualities, those aspects of our "self" that are intrinsic and perhaps, or at least historically, immutable. Along this path, questions about the origins of health and disease tend to focus inward, on the *nature* of the healthy and the sick, and

Environmental Biodynamics. Manish Arora and Paul Curtin with Austen Curtin, Christine Austin, and Alessandro Giuliani, Oxford University Press. © Oxford University Press 2022. DOI: 10.1093/oso/9780197582947.003.0002

how that nature is inherited. This notion of inheritance has been with us for as long as we have records of human existence and has of course been extended beyond just our physical features to the often-lamentable hierarchies in the organization of our societies.

The second path these questions follow tends to focus outward, instead, on the *exogenous* origins of health and disease. Rather than ask what of our health is inherited, this path focuses on how health and disease are *nurtured* in us by our environment. This perspective, too, has been with us from our beginnings, from the specification of diets for the young, the old, the pregnant, and so on, and in the use of herbs and early medicines for the treatment of disease (and, conversely, in the use of poisons to inflict disease).

In the past century we have seen the emergence of new technologies that have vastly enhanced our capabilities to study the origins of health and disease both internally and externally. Curiously, the advent of genomic technologies, which for the first time allowed us to trace at large scale the inherited mechanisms of disease, and the proliferation of precise chemical sensors and biomonitoring technologies to identify and characterize aspects of the environment that may impact our health, have not yielded a triumphant validation of either perspective. Instead, a third path has become the prevalent view in medicine and biology—that it is in the integration of internal *and* external factors upon which health and disease are predicated. Certainly, our genes play a role in our vulnerability to disease, but it is through environmental exposures that the effects of these propensities become evident in our health; and, vice versa, that our genes act in a background of environmentally determined predisposition. For example, an inherited inability to metabolize cow milk is only relevant in an environment that includes dairy farming.

This third view, the "gene-by-environment" perspective (often referred to as G × E), has become the predominant view in modern medicine on the origins of health and disease, and in fact one can expect to hear our risks for a given disease commonly expressed in these terms. At the time of writing this book, the risk of developing autism spectrum disorder (ASD), for example, is thought to be driven 50% to 80% by genetics and approximately 20% to 50% by environmental factors.[1] But in the past decade, it has become increasingly apparent that while the integration of environment and genes is essential to understanding both inherited and acquired health characteristics, it is certainly not sufficient to explain *health*. In this book, we offer a fourth path—that for a more comprehensive understanding of how the external environment interacts with our internal physiology, we must consider functional dynamics, which manifest in the organization of time-dependent change. It is our view that *time* is the crucial missing piece in the current worldview of health and disease.

Structuralism, Reductionism, and Simplicity

In many aspects of science, and especially in medicine, we perceive the world through the lens of "thingness." By this we mean that medical science has become entrenched in thinking of our physiology and our environment as a collection of things that are connected in certain ways. *Structuralism*, which is the school of thought underlying this worldview, analyzes a system through the composition of its parts; an anatomical study, for example. *Reductionism*, likewise, posits that the best way to scientifically understand a system is to investigate it by fragmenting it into smaller pieces.[1] This is accompanied by the notion that any complexity observed in nature can be explained by examining its components at a finer scale. An enduring appeal in these perspectives is that, as with any good idea, they tell us what to look for, in particular in our investigation of human health. To better understand our physiology, we must simply examine our anatomy at ever-smaller spatial scales from organs to cells to molecules; and, likewise, to understand our environment we must analyze its constituent parts.

The almost universal embrace of reductionist perspectives in studies on human health has had broader implications beyond the questions of what to measure; it has also impacted how we ask questions and what answers we accept as truths. For example, in characterizing the endogenous origins of disease, the reductionist paradigm leads us to identify the structural properties of our physiology, and link these to our health; similarly, in considering the role of the environment, we reduce our climate, neighborhood, diet, and workspace to its constituent parts, and seek to link those components to our health.

---

[1] For a more thorough and in-depth discussion of these concepts, see the wonderful *Beyond Mechanism:Putting Life Back into Biology* by Brian G. Henning and Adam C. Scarfe (Lanham, MD: Lexington Books, 2013).

Box 2.1 Historical Aside

How did structuralism and reductionism become so pervasive in medicine? There are many places this story could begin, from Aristotle through Descartes, but for the present discussion, let us consider the advent of microbiology. In the 1670s, Antonie Philips van Leeuwenhoek, a Dutch drapery maker who was also a self-taught lens maker and scientist, made a rudimentary single-lens microscope with which he observed microbes, red blood cells, and many other microscopic components of living organisms. Around the same time English philosopher Robert Hooke coined the term "cell" to describe the honeycomb-like patterns he had seen under a simple microscope. Subsequently, scientists identified cells of different types and then the nucleus as the control center of the cell and intracellular organelles that served various purposes. Now the most sensitive microscopes can reveal single atoms.

This approach of examining ever-smaller components persists in modern medicine, and environmental medicine is no exception. For example, the discovery of DNA and the subsequent advent of genetics, which led to the Human Genome Project's mapping of the entire human genetic sequence, has resulted in an unprecedented effort to use genetics to solve the biggest problems facing human health. As microscopy enabled us to describe the spatial structure of our cells, genetics revealed a "code" to describe the blueprint for the traits that supposedly favored health or disease. Once the structure of DNA was characterized using protein chemistry methods, we had these "things"—genes—that we thought could explain every aspect of our physiology. And we approached genes as if they were immutable objects; in fact, we made them so static that we described them with combinations of structural building blocks known by just four letters (a, g, c, and t, which stand for the nucleotides adenine, guanine, cytosine, and thymine). We are not criticizing genetics, and, to be fair, there has been some success using genetics. For example, several serious disorders have been linked to mutations in our genes.[2] However, genomics has fallen far short of explaining as many aspects of human health and disease as originally hoped; in fact, it explains a very small proportion of the diseases that are the major causes of death.[3]

Reductionism and structural thinking are also pervasive in environmental health and related fields. "The dose makes the poison" has been a central dogma for toxicology for centuries, but this sole focus on intensity or dose excludes the dynamics of environmental influences. Throughout this book we will give examples where a shift from a purely structural to a functional view of the environment gave us new insight and helped us develop tools to better understand human health and disease.

Consider what these associations imply through the lens of complexity, as outlined through the perspective of Warren Weaver in Chapter 1. Structuralist and reductionist paradigms inevitably lead to a scientific worldview embedded in two notions—that of *organized simplicity*, whereby two systems directly influence one another, or that of *disorganized complexity*, whereby many variables may be involved but all are ultimately related through a construct of group-level averages. This framework arises as an inevitable consequence of the static, dichotomized nature of how we consider the complex systems involved in human health. Rather than a *physiological* view of human health, which would comprise dynamic, time-varying systems of embedded processes, reductionism diminishes human physiology, and the environment it emerges in, to a static, anatomical or molecular perspective. In that context of fixed, static measurements, the interdependent processes that give rise to *organized complexity* (Weaver's third realm of complexity) are inaccessible. According to Environmental Biodynamics, complex systems such as the environment and human physiology interact through the action of interdependent processes *over time*. The limitations inherent in contemporary practices by which we design and implement environmental health studies, and the answers we have so far arrived at, which are woefully incomplete, are something that we seek to overcome.

A Puzzle for You

To understand how reductionist thinking and current epidemiological paradigms limit our understanding of complex systems, we ask the reader to consider the following hypothetical. We want you to assume the role of a scientist in this story we are about to tell. It is the story of experiments undertaken at four different laboratories to study the same system. At the end of this exercise, you are asked to answer two questions:

1. What is the underlying system?
2. Which laboratory adopted the best perspective to study the underlying system?

We need to lay down some ground rules because we want you to realize that no environmental epidemiological study has infinite resources or access to some magical technology that can remove unforeseen barriers as they arise. Scientists also have to make judgment calls about the study's design at the beginning of a study, and often changing course midway is not an option. For example, we are part of studies that undertake environmental exposure measurements and health assessments on thousands of participants repeatedly at regular intervals of time. We had to decide on many logistical design issues at the beginning; for instance:

- *How often would the participants come back to the study headquarters for their assessments?* We decided once a year, because more frequent visits would make the study prohibitively expensive.
- *How long would each visit last?* We decided on four to five hours, because our study includes children, and keeping them and their parents for longer would be too arduous and likely deter them from being part of the study. This decision in turn limited how many medical assessments we could undertake.

There are many other realities of epidemiological studies, but by now, we hope you can appreciate that conducting studies on humans requires careful compromise and tough decisions driven by, among other things, logistics. There is never an option to measure everything at every possible spatial and temporal resolution.

Now, let's begin. You are asked to observe a system for which you have no prior information. We will set some parameters for the experiment; these are the tough decisions we mentioned earlier that every scientist has to make at the start of a study. You have resources for five consecutive measurements, and the total time period for which you can keep this study going is 10 units of time (it could be months, years, or some other timespan, but for this example let's make it 10 seconds). The measurements are instantaneous observations of the system's state, like examining a cell under a microscope, studying a star through a telescope, or doing a blood test—that is, they are like snapshots, and it is so because your technology only allows that. Again, this mimics reality in that epidemiologists can only use the technology available to them.

We present four different scenarios under which the experiment could be conducted; of course, there are many other options too and you are free to reconstruct the experiment under different parameters, but you must always follow the rules—only five consecutive instantaneous measurements over a total timespan of 10 seconds. Table 2.1 contains the results at the different labs, which we'll summarize here—but by all means read the data and come to your own conclusions. Scientists at Lab 1 decide that they will spread their measurements over two-second intervals starting at Time 1. At Lab 2, the decision was to do the same but start at Time 2. In Lab 3, the scientists observed the system at one-second intervals starting at Time 1. Lab 4 decided to go

Table 2.1 Results of Experiments at Different Laboratories

Lab 1		Lab 2		Lab 3		Lab 4	
Time	Result	Time	Result	Time	Result	Time	Result
1	● Dark	2	○ Bright	1	● Dark	1.1	● Dark
3	● Dark	4	○ Bright	2	○ Bright	1.2	● Dark
5	● Dark	6	○ Bright	3	● Dark	1.3	● Dark
7	● Dark	8	○ Bright	4	○ Bright	1.4	● Dark
9	● Dark	10	○ Bright	5	● Dark	1.5	● Dark
Interpretation of results	- No signal detected; field of view is empty		- Bright light observed at all times - System has only one stationary state		- Two stationary states detected; bright and dark		- No signal detected; field of view is empty

with the finest temporal resolution available and observe the system at 0.1-second intervals. In the bottom row, we give the interpretation of the findings reached at each lab.

Having reviewed the results, what do you believe you are looking at? And which laboratory do you think adopted the best temporal resolution? Or, would you have adopted an entirely different temporal resolution? In the next paragraph, we reveal the underlying truth, but please keep in mind that in reality the underlying truth is never revealed to us. There is no such thing in science as absolute certainty or a complete answer with no missing information. We asked some of our friends and colleagues from different walks of life to attempt this puzzle, and the most common answer we received was that the system we are observing is a light that alternates between being on and off; that is, Lab 3 came out the winner.

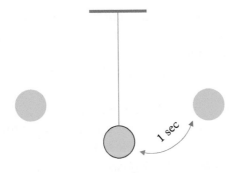

Left (not visible to experimenter)	Center (visible to experimenter)	Right (not visible to experimenter)
1	0	3
5	2	7
9	4	11
13	6	15
17	8	19

Figure 2.1 The points when the pendulum is at each position. The pendulum is visible to the experimenter only at the center position.

Here is a description of what the underlying system actually is. It is a frictionless pendulum with a glowing disc at the end; through the lens of the sampling instrument, which we defined as some sort of scope, the experimenter observes the system when it is at its center state. The pendulum takes a second to travel from the center position to the farthest positions on the left or right of center. The time points when the pendulum is at each location are shown in Figure 2.1. You can appreciate that the observer, who is aligned with the center position, only sees the pendulum's disc for an instant when it is at the center every two seconds. This is why to the observer it appears as a light that flashes in two-second cycles.

For those of you who had guessed that the system is a flashing light or even a rotating disc that has a bright light on one side and is dark on the other, you are not wrong. In fact, there are other options that would be indistinguishable under the given conditions. But take a moment to appreciate the difference between the pendulum and the flashing light scenarios. Under the flashing light scenario, the scientists at Lab 3 have perfect prediction, but they consider the system to be static, when it is not. In reality, the system is always in the "on" position, but to the scientists it appears to be alternating between "on" and "off."

The lesson here is that how we perceive a system is dependent on our scalar perspective! Returning to the general question of human environment and health that is the main focus of this book, we must now ask: *How have the scales of our measurements constrained our understanding of environment–human interactions?*

The example we have just presented may appear highly contrived, and it admittedly is, but the fundamental limitations here are exactly the same as in so many studies investigating human–environment interactions, especially observational epidemiological studies. In fact, this experiment would also pass the test of replication if another laboratory undertook measurements under similar conditions. Just because the experimental results can be repeated doesn't make them any more accurate in this example.

So, how do we overcome these limitations? At present we set the timing of visits at intervals that are designed for logistical reasons. For example, while attending a recent planning meeting to include the gut microbiome in an established prospective cohort study, it was decided that the participants would bring a stool sample when they come in for their annual study visit to the study headquarters (this visit is when a whole range of medical tests are done). The reasons given to justify this plan were all logistical—the complexity of shipping the samples at other times, the expense of more frequent sample collection and analysis, and so on. Our point is not that these considerations are unimportant, but that they cannot be where the discussion starts. Instead, the first step should be to identify a scale of measurement that allows us to explore the dynamics of the system we are studying. As in our example, this will likely require initial stages of trial and error; but, as illustrated, we will know the appropriate scale when we begin to see insights into the underlying *temporal dynamics* in the system we are interested in.

We propose that environmental health studies incorporate an initial pilot phase designed specifically to explore the temporal dynamics of the systems under investigation. In our microbiome example, the question to ask is this: What is the temporal resolution over which the microbiome changes within the context of the main study hypotheses? At this point, many good epidemiologists will be thinking that often we do not know what the appropriate temporal resolution is at the start of the study. That is an excellent point and an accurate reflection of the challenges of research on humans. The approach we recommend is that when undertaking the pilot phase, it is important to vary the temporal resolution. For example, if in our experiment of the flashing light and the pendulum, we had taken measurements that included the timepoints 2.1 and 2.2 seconds (or 1.8, 1.9, and many other possible options), then our data would have shown that the pendulum no longer occupies the whole field of view and a small crescent of darkness appears and grows bigger with the passage of time (a picture akin to the phases of the moon). This would then prompt us to redesign our experiment to capture the onset and end of these dynamics and, in subsequent experiments, to identify the persistence of these effects, the mechanisms that maintain them, and the process by which this system came to a stable dynamic. This reflects a profound reorganization of inquiry in environmental health and medicine, with the focus switching from the examination of static relationships to the exploration of temporal dynamics.

Environmental Biodynamics: Rethinking the Role of Time in Environmental Health Research

The same structural and reductionist thinking that prevented some of our hypothetical laboratories from unraveling the nature of the system they were observing also restricts current approaches in environmental health research to the domains of organized simplicity and disorganized complexity. Why are current approaches not able to leverage organized complexity? To answer this, and to recognize the role of Environmental Biodynamics in overcoming this limitation, we must take a critical look at some contemporary methods of environmental health data collection. Let's start with how we design our research studies, but note this explanation is intended as a high-level survey, which inevitably paints with a broad brush.[2]

When it comes to recruiting participants into a study and collecting data on their environment and their health, many highly regarded studies in environmental epidemiology adopt a longitudinal design, most often a prospective

---

[2] For detailed explanations of current standards in epidemiological study design, interested readers may wish to consider the excellent text *Modern Epidemiology* (4th edition) by Timothy L. Lash, Tyler J. VanderWeele, Sebastien Haneause, and Kenneth Rothman (Wolters Kluwer, 2020; ISBN-10: 9781451190052).

cohort approach. There are many reasons for this that are beyond the scope of this book; any basic textbook on environmental epidemiology will shed light on that topic as well as provide formal definitions of different study designs such as *cohort studies, case-control studies, randomized trials,* and others.

In the simplest terms, *cohort* refers to a group of participants recruited into a study based on shared characteristics and examined under similar conditions.[3] A *prospective* study is one where we collect data on our participants at intervals of time moving forward. For example, we, the authors, are interested in how environmental factors during pregnancy can impact the child's life, so we have initiated several pregnancy cohort studies. In these efforts, we request women participants to volunteer into our study when they are first aware of being pregnant, and then we begin to collect measures of environmental exposures (diet, air pollution, toxic chemicals in blood, as a few examples from a very long list of measures). We also collect health data at regular intervals (usually six months to one year) ranging from anthropometric measurements (body weight, blood pressure, and many others) to clinical measures of ill health (diabetes, asthma, etc.). We collect similar measurements on their babies. Importantly, we "bank" blood, urine, and other biological samples in freezers so that we can analyze them at a future date.

Why do we do this repeated collection of data? Again, there are many reasons that are discussed in epidemiology textbooks, but the foremost is to resolve the "chicken-and-egg" problem. We want to be able to measure environmental exposures *before* the onset of illness so that we can establish if the exposure of interest increases the risk of disease, and it wasn't a case where the disease caused an increase in exposure. For example, studies have shown that levels of the toxic metal lead are elevated in children who receive diagnoses for autism—but, to verify that lead exposure is indeed involved in the etiology of the disease, it is important to measure lead exposure *before* the onset of the clinical signs of ASD to establish the correct temporal order, because the reverse is also possible.[4–7] For example, children with autism have an increased tendency to put non-food items from the floor in their mouths (this habit is known as *pica*), which can increase their lead exposure; in other words, the behavioral traits of autism can cause an increase in how much lead enters your body.

---

[3] Those interested in a more in-depth description of a prospective cohort study design can refer to the *Dictionary of Epidemiology* and other standard texts of epidemiology.

But this approach of measuring the suspected cause or risk factors before the onset of clinical disease is not the same as measuring temporal dynamics. To convey this point, we highlight three shortcomings in current epidemiological approaches that must be overcome if we are to truly incorporate *time* into environmental health research and advance this very important scientific field.

First, we must recognize that undertaking a prospective cohort study that takes measurements on the participants and their environment at regular intervals falls short of uncovering the true temporal nature of our physiology and our environment. The typical longitudinal study design aims to test a hypothesis at multiple timepoints—for example, in our own studies we have measured lead exposure at different ages (at birth and then at 12 and 18 months of age) and then we correlated each of these measures with later cognitive performance.[7] This is nothing but a structural analysis repeated at multiple timepoints and should not be mistaken for a functional assessment. In stark contrast, Environmental Biodynamics seeks to characterize the temporal dynamics that serve as an interface between the environmental exposure (lead, in this case) and our physiology. While both approaches inevitably include repeated assessments of lead exposure, the appropriate scale of those measurements differs tremendously. In the prospective cohort study the scale of those measurements is driven often by logistics—participants are called in once a year to the study headquarters (often a hospital or clinic where medical equipment is available), and consequently their health and environment are measured once a year, whereas a study focused on temporal dynamics will require a sampling resolution that is scaled according to the *function* of the system under study. As such, and as in our earlier example of the pendulum, the scale of these measurements must be appropriate to capture change in these systems. Think of it like this—to understand how a hummingbird flaps its wings, an hourly measurement would be too coarse, but to study its sleep habits, an hourly measurement would provide useful information. In the same manner, to capture dynamics relevant to metabolism on a weekly or monthly timescale might require daily measurements; to capture circadian (daily) dynamics, hourly samples might be required.

The second shortcoming of current epidemiological approaches has been in the way we analyze our data. By now, some savvy epidemiologists would have argued against the first point, citing examples of studies that collect repeated measures of biomarkers—for example, the collection of cortisol every few hours to examine stress events (cortisol is a hormone linked with states of heightened excitement). While these approaches have improved the temporal resolution of the sampling procedure, they typically fall short of uncovering dynamics because of the way the data are analyzed.

The conventional approach in these and other longitudinal or repeated-measures studies is to construct a modeling strategy that links the magnitude of the exposure or variable of interest—here, cortisol—to some health outcome, while controlling for time. These approaches, typically achieved through statistical methods (for example, mixed-effect modeling, a term referring to an array of statistical techniques), control for repeated measurements in time, but they are not typically leveraged to analyze the dynamics of change over time; rather, *time* is merely treated as nuisance variable while some other relationship is evaluated in earnest. Though this critique admittedly paints the field with a very broad brush, and we would note as well that several groups have developed innovative methods to leverage time more effectively (again, savvy epidemiologists would recognize methods such as distributed lag models, latent trajectory analysis, and more sophisticated implementations of linear and non-linear mixed-effect modeling), our field does not treat temporal dynamics as an endpoint in itself. In contrast, the implementation of a functional perspective treats the dynamics over time as the fundamental measure of interest and considers the individual momentary measures as merely contributing to the overall dynamic.

The third challenge we face in environmental epidemiology is that we have falsely ascended *associations* to be the fundamental method of connecting one system to another. In essence, this implies that a change in one variable relates to a change in another variable, which is certainly a meaningful and intuitive measure of a relationship. But this is unambiguously not the *only* meaningful dependency that might be of biomedical interest and should certainly not be the entirety of scientific focus. Other patterns that should equally be the focus of biomedical enquiry include the investigation of rhythms and other periodic dynamics: chaotic behavior, the transfer of information from one system to another, reciprocal dynamics, and interdependencies. Perhaps most profoundly, we have ignored the idea that there are fundamental rules that organize a given system.

It is clear that to overcome these limitations requires us to rethink the design of our epidemiological studies, but beyond that we also need to develop new technologies to measure environmental and biological systems at better temporal resolutions, and better approaches to analyzing data that embrace the *organized complexity* of the systems under study.

Box 2.2 On the Nature of Time and Change

We have discussed *time* and *dynamics* (change over time) throughout this chapter and will do so intermittently throughout the book. This then raises an obvious question: How are "time" and "change" related? The idea that time is intrinsically linked with change was discussed as early as the fourth century BCE by Aristotle in Book IV of *Physics*. Time has been measured by observing changes in sun clocks, sand (hourglass), water, even candles, and currently the most advanced technologies to measure time rely on atomic decay. However, the main way we humans perceive time is through its entanglement with change. The study of human health and disease is more about what changes (and when and how change occurs) and less about what stays the same. For example, when we say that we all age with time, we are essentially saying we change over time. Does every part of our body, at every scale of measurement, change at the same rate? Obviously not. During the past year, not only has our body as a whole changed (aged), but many of the body's components, our tissues and organs, have also changed. Skin cells are renewed every 21 days or so, and red blood cells are replaced about every four months. Even our chromosomes have changed; the telomere length is now shorter than it was a year ago. The pathways that metabolize the components of our food and affect whether our body gains or loses weight also change. However, when we examine the physiological changes associated with aging at ever-finer scales, we come to an important paradoxical realization: The atoms (and the subatomic particles that compose them) that build the molecules that form the cells that function as our tissues and organs—these building blocks of matter do not age.[a] The atoms and their subatomic components are the same as they were a year ago, and they will be the same next year. This is a profound aspect of our reality that begs a profound question: *How do different systems operating across vastly different timescales—some, like subatomic particles, not changing, others. like neurons. firing at milliseconds. and some operating over months—function in unison?*

Incorporating Biodynamics and the Shape of Change into Population Health

The points raised in the prior section emphasize two essential truths with regard to current epidemiological study design. First, far too many contemporary perspectives in environmental medicine embrace a static, reductionist assessment of environmental health that implicitly assumes a system of *disorganized complexity*; rather than explain complexity at the level of the

---

[a] In reality atoms age as well through the process of atomic decay, but that extends over many centuries rather than the timescale of a human life, and electrons and protons do not decay and therefore do not age.

individual, it focuses on the statistical derivation of population norms, and relates these norms to health. A second, more pernicious implication is that the pervasive reliance of group-level correlations is implicitly incapable of considering homeostasis and dynamics at the level of the individual. Precision environmental medicine then falls outside the scope of a majority of studies and hampers their translation to clinical practice.

To clarify these points, we will use data from a large and highly regarded study. The U.S. National Health and Nutrition Examination Survey (NHANES) is a nationwide study that measures the health of U.S. residents from multiple geographical locations in the country. It is so nicely designed that the results represent the entire nation of 300 million people. During the study, thousands of participants from all ages and backgrounds are enrolled into the study in a systematic manner and data on their demographics (age, ethnic backgrounds, income, education level, and many other factors) are recorded. Blood and urine samples are collected for testing and a detailed medical exam is performed as well. And yes, environmental exposures are also measured by testing the blood and urine for markers of various chemicals, recording diet on a questionnaire, and asking questions about active and passive smoking. The goal of this effort is to provide health and environmental exposure assessments that reflect the entire nation's population and, although subjects are not tracked longitudinally, to provide an indicator of how these factors change in the population over successive rounds of the survey.

For our present discussion, we will use blood zinc levels from the 2014 NHANES. From these we can derive the distribution of zinc levels (and the associated probability density function), as shown in Figure 2.2, which tells us how probable it is (Y-axis) that any individual will have a given zinc level (X-axis). In this context, the blood zinc level of an individual is defined as healthy if it falls between the 2.5th percentile (in this case, 58 µg/dL) and the 97.5th percentile (115 µg/dL). The 2.5th to 97.5th percentile cutoff limits are based on age-old rules of thumb and are now widely used for many physiological parameters. In current clinical practice, a patient's blood zinc level would be compared to this graph.

This appears perfectly reasonable and intuitive from both medical and scientific perspectives. To understand how zinc relates to health, a scientist could simply relate zinc levels to some measured outcome—for example, we could ask whether, as body weight increases, one's location on this curve changes. If this happens in a consistent manner, then we can conclude that body weight and zinc are correlated. Similarly, from the perspective of environmental

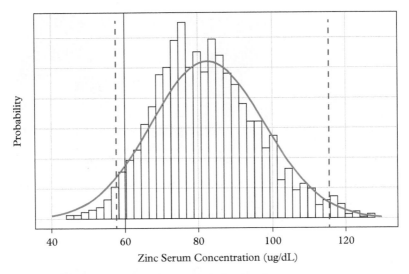

Figure 2.2 U.S. population norms for blood zinc level.

Data from National Health and Nutrition Examination Survey Data. Centers for Disease Control and Prevention (CDC). National Center for Health Statistics (NCHS).

medicine, these distributions provide a standard to assess an individual's "level" of zinc exposure: Are their "levels" too high, too low, or "just right"? It seems that the perspective of disorganized complexity does have its uses—but of course, in both applications, there is a catch.

The problem here emerges prior to the applications just described, or in the details of the cohort study design: It is in the assumption of a static, structural interpretation of zinc levels. Contrary to these conceptions, zinc does not simply "hold still" like some static constant; rather, it varies throughout the day in concert with other biological dynamics (often referred to as "rhythms," but that is misleading since rhythms are not the only type of dynamics our physiology exhibits). A seminal study by Wendy Scales and colleagues at the University of Michigan elegantly demonstrated this process.[8] Rather than measure zinc levels at a single time in a huge population, as in NHANES, they repeatedly measured blood zinc levels of a few healthy subjects at four-hour intervals. The results, as shown in Figure 2.3, revealed that zinc levels fluctuate throughout the day in a rhythmic pattern following our circadian rhythm. In the morning, zinc levels started to increase, reaching their peak around 8 a.m., and then began to decrease, reaching their lowest levels in the late afternoon and early evening. Closer examination of the range in zinc levels indicates a span, on average, from approximately 65 µg/dL at its lowest

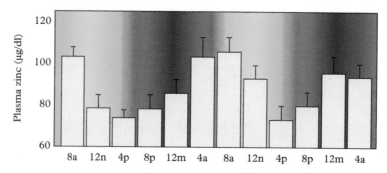

Figure 2.3 Blood zinc levels over the span of two days (modified from the study by Scales and colleagues[8]). Concentrations reach their peak of between 100 and 110 μg/dL around 8 a.m. and are at their lowest around 4 p.m.

12m = midnight, 12n = noon.

point to 110 μg/dL at its highest. You will notice that the range within a single individual over the course of a day is roughly similar to the range of the population average as revealed in NHANES. This is not a coincidence. What is happening is that, unbeknownst to the users of the NHANES data, the survey is very much behaving like the laboratories in our example of the pendulum and the flashing light: It is reporting a static range of values for a dynamic system.

The implications of this for precision medicine are profound. Consider an individual that, upon visiting their physician's office, has their blood sample analyzed to characterize the levels of essential elements. The sample is drawn at 4:30 p.m., and when the results are returned their blood zinc level is 90 μg/dL. Under a static structural view embedded in disorganized complexity—such as comparing the patient's blood test results to the NHANES data—this number is within the normal range of 58 to 115 μg/dL, and we would consider this person to be healthy in regard to this one metric. But when we reconsider the temporal biodynamics of zinc homeostasis, realizing that 4 p.m. is actually the low point for zinc rhythms, when blood zinc should be around 65 μg/dL, the patient is actually well outside the normal range.

Clinicians and researchers are not entirely insensitive to these dynamics and challenges in exposure assessment and will be quick to point out that, for these very reasons, many diagnostic tests are performed at certain times of the day, with specific restrictions imposed, such as fasting. And, indeed, these measures can be useful in controlling for functional dynamics in homeostatic processes, such as rhythms. However, while these procedures may *control* for temporal dynamics, they are failing to leverage and analyze them, leaving critical physiological questions unasked.

To convey how important physiological processes may be overlooked by traditional structural reductionism, consider the hypothetical prospective study shown in Figure 2.4. In this study, blood zinc was measured once every day for four days. In panel A we show the results of three individuals viewed from a purely structural perspective, with each subject's measures indicated by a different color. All three subjects are within a "normal" range and might superficially appear healthy. However, given what we know about the periodicity of zinc from the study by Scales and colleagues, there is more to homeostasis than a momentary concentration, and we can leverage this information to predict where concentrations should be when based on functional dynamics. In panel B, when we superimpose the expected circadian rhythm for the "blue" subject, we see that their measurements perfectly correspond to the expected dynamic cycle. In panels C and D, however, when we make the same projections for the gray and red subjects, we see the emergence of different potential abnormalities (unhealthy states) that would be wrongly classified as normal by the structural approach. The gray dotted line shows that the daily rhythm of blood zinc levels has undergone a phase shift—it peaks earlier in the morning. The red line is initially further phase-shifted and then shows a complete loss of rhythm in the third and fourth days (i.e., a flat signal). Both the gray and red profiles are showing signs of deviation from a healthy zinc profile, but that one blood test we have done once a year as part of our annual physical would not pick up this early warning alarm.

Consider the contrast between this hypothetical study and the examination of zinc homeostasis through a structural perspective, as in NHANES. Whereas the disorganized complexity of the zinc distributions at the level of the population was the focus of the structural perspective in NHANES, the new *functional* perspective offered by Environmental Biodynamics focuses on the organized complexity in the dynamics of zinc homeostasis. From a structural perspective, what matters is the purportedly static "level" of the environmental exposure; but, from a functional perspective, the focus is on the organization of the exposure in the dimension of *time*, in this case a rhythmic process. Here, we would like to take you back to the example of the pendulum and the four laboratories that undertook snapshot experiments, very much embedded in a structural perspective. When concluding that section, we had said that the experiment was contrived, but now that we have discussed the dynamics of zinc, we have seen that in many ways our zinc metabolism

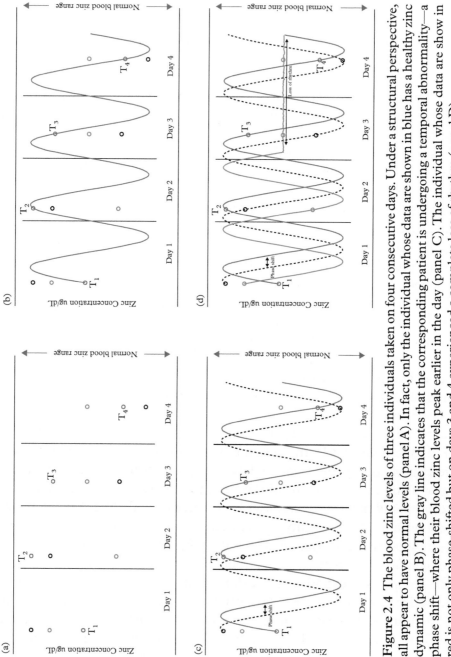

Figure 2.4 The blood zinc levels of three individuals taken on four consecutive days. Under a structural perspective, all appear to have normal levels (panel A). In fact, only the individual whose data are shown in blue has a healthy zinc dynamic (panel B). The gray line indicates that the corresponding patient is undergoing a temporal abnormality—a phase shift—where their blood zinc levels peak earlier in the day (panel C). The individual whose data are show in red is not only phase-shifted but on days 3 and 4 experienced a complete loss of rhythm (panel D).

behaves very much like a pendulum—in fact, the sine wave form of the zinc levels over a day shown in Figures 2.3 and 2.4 is exactly the same as the sine wave formed by the path of a pendulum.

What we have learned so far is that the focus of Environmental Biodynamics is to advance, develop, and implement functional perspectives in environmental health sciences and to leverage these to bring new insights to the practice of environmental medicine. This approach depends on the properties of both the organism and the environment, as both constantly vary over time. By studying the nature of these time-varying processes, rather than momentary states, a functional perspective leverages measures of dynamic properties in ways that the structural perspective does not. That is, measures of intensity or velocity at the wrong scale are insufficient to characterize human development and function.[4] Neither regularities nor irregularities can be appreciated in a static view of human physiology. Hence, Environmental Biodynamics recognizes that human development and function are not linear processes but are a product of high-dimensional overlapping and interacting dynamics.

A Hard Lesson to Learn: Repeated Structural Analyses Do Not Equal a Functional Interpretation (Case Study)

Studies like those by Scales and colleagues have long paved the way for functional approaches to environmental health and medicine, but serious challenges have stood in the way of implementing these in routine medical practice. Foremost among these is the formidable challenge of collecting repeated measurements from the same person. This will always present a serious logistical hurdle—being told to visit your doctor 10 times instead of once will never go over well—but can also present physiological challenges, for example if the tissue analyzed is vital, ephemeral, or in limited supply. However, for all the difficulties these issues present, our experience in developing functional approaches is that there are still deeper challenges than in the data collection.

The critical advance that made all our efforts in developing a functional perspective possible, from which we extend the field of Environmental Biodynamics, was the development of a technology that allowed us to obtain

---

[4] We recognize that technological advances will need to occur in order to fully implement the functional perspective. See the appendix for the technologies we have used.

data at multiple timepoints all from a single sample, as if looking at a series of time capsules (we refer to these as *retrospective temporal exposure biomarkers*). This technology is described in the appendix, but to describe it in general terms, it suffices to say that it leverages the remarkable, and for us the terribly convenient, biology of tooth development. An amazing fact about deciduous teeth (i.e., "baby" teeth) is that they start forming before we are born, so whenever children shed their baby teeth, they are providing us with a repository of their exposures from the second trimester through the age when the tooth was shed. Another interesting point about teeth is that they form growth rings, like trees do, so, much like a fallen tree, one can trace the patterns in the growth rings to identify the timing of critical life events. Our laboratory developed an approach whereby we apply fine laser beams to systematically map the growth rings in shed baby teeth and, using targeted mass spectrometry, measure chemical concentrations along these growth trajectories. This allows us to build a timeline of chemical exposures starting in the second trimester into childhood—from a single tooth sample, hundreds of repeated measurements can be obtained. In contrast to the blood tests that have been discussed thus far, which provide momentary snapshots of chemical exposures at one discrete moment, this retrospective biomarker allows us to analyze the history of chemical exposures throughout development. To put this in context, a blood test for the toxic metal lead only provides information on how much you were exposed to over the last few months, but an analysis of teeth can answer the seemingly impossible question of how much lead you were exposed to before you were born. These tools provide an amazing opportunity to answer important questions about the role of environmental inputs in human development. By collecting and analyzing shed baby teeth, we can assess not just the magnitude of exposures but also their *timing* in gestation and early childhood.

Next, to provide a concrete example of how *time* has been incorporated into the structural approach in epidemiological research, we describe an early ASD study of ours. By sharing this and our subsequent studies, we will build a bridge that takes the reader over that most important of chasms, the one from theory to clinical practice. We also want to be free to criticize practices that fail to incorporate functional perspectives, and there is no better place in science to be critical than of your own work. Along the way, you will learn many things about ASD and our exposure to nutritional and toxic metals. That is not the purpose of the book, but having an actual health-related example that we can use throughout the book helps us convey the utility of the theory to actual medical practice.

This initial study that we will describe, prior to our work on Environmental Biodynamics, relied entirely on a structural approach. We provide a summary of that study here, and all technical aspects can be found in our journal article.[7] We wanted to determine whether children with autism metabolized trace metals differently than children without autism. This topic was chosen in response to several prior studies that showed that autistic children had higher blood levels of some toxic metals, such as lead, or lower levels of essential nutrients, such as zinc. Most of those studies were plagued by a major problem: The biomarkers for the elements and compounds being studied were measured *after* autism had been diagnosed. Consequently, there was a chicken-and-egg problem: We could not be sure whether the imbalances in these essential and toxic elements themselves caused autism or, conversely, were a downstream consequence of the pathological processes associated with autism. In other words, does the pathology underlying the autism spectrum result in more lead being consumed? That was indeed possible, because it is known that children with autism exhibit signs of pica, a condition in which children eat non-food items, which could then increase their chances of ingesting more lead from dirt and house dust.[5]

Second, we suspected that whatever was driving the development of autism might be present prenatally; that is, an environmental exposure during gestation might be linked to the emergence of autism in childhood. The problem that we faced was this: For the children we were studying, some of whom had ASD and some of whom did not, how do we go back in time and measure their fetal metabolism? It would be too dangerous to conduct a prospective study and collect fetal blood during gestation, and maternal levels of metals in blood do not always reflect fetal levels accurately (because the placenta regulates what passes from the mother to the fetus for many environmental exposures). Readers can ask themselves this question too: *Do you know precisely what environmental chemicals you were exposed to before you were born?*

There was one more issue. We knew that autism has a genetic component. At the time we undertook the study, estimates of heritability ranged from 50% to 80%, which meant that we must account for genetic influences in addition to the environmental and non-genetic signals. To have a handle on the genetic

---

[5] See the Centers for Disease Control and Prevention's website for the most common sources of lead in children's environments: https://www.cdc.gov/nceh/lead/prevention/sources.htm.

factors, we undertook the study in a group of Swedish twins in which one twin had autism and the other did not. Because twins have similar genetic sequences, and in the case of monozygotic twins the genetic sequences are almost identical, twin studies are a powerful tool to compare the contribution of environmental and genetic factors in disease risk. To go back in time to measure fetal exposures, we used the technology relying on shed deciduous ("baby") teeth that we described earlier. This method allows us to look at fetal and early childhood uptake of several elements (essential nutrients and toxic metals) at week-by-week resolution.

It is a rare privilege to work at the confluence of such complementary study designs and technologies, and consequently we approached the analysis of these data with great enthusiasm. Our colleague in Sweden, Dr. Sven Bölte, who heads a major neurodevelopmental research center at the Karolinska Institute in Stockholm, met with the children for comprehensive diagnostic and clinical assessments and duly provided us with the children's shed teeth for analysis. We approached these with the finest-scale analyses we were capable of, eager to uncover potentially subtle temporal dynamics and interactions. And, when all was said and done, we had created what we sought to achieve—a comprehensive map of chemical exposures in each child that traced from their second trimester through their first year of life. In particular, our analysis focused on essential elements such as zinc and copper that our body needs in the right amount to maintain health and nonessential (i.e., generally toxic) metals such as lead that are harmful to us even at very low levels.

These results preceded, but ultimately paved the way for, the functional perspective we would later develop into Environmental Biodynamics, but at the time we implemented a sophisticated albeit standard structural analysis of these data. This was done through a type of statistical method called a distributed lag model, which uses tests for associations between time-series data and a health outcome—in our case, between chemical exposure trajectories and ASD diagnosis. The method allowed us to identify not just *if* chemical exposures related to ASD but also *when*, in the child's development, the exposure relates to ASD. Continuing this chapter's use of zinc homeostasis as an example, here we share some insights into the role of this essential element in ASD.

While we measured over a dozen essential nutrients and toxic metals, the results for zinc really stood out. Zinc is an essential part of our nutrition. It is a key component of several hundred enzymes in our body, and it participates in pathways that play a role in various functions, ranging from regulation of the immune system to digesting food to reproduction. Figure 2.5 compares weekly zinc levels between twins who had autism and their siblings who did not. The graph in Figure 2.5 arises from rather technical data that will only be familiar to those who are routinely using time-series data. We have, therefore, adapted a simpler figure, but the original can be found in our journal article.[7] The blue band indicates the nature of the relationship (the correlation, in a sense) between zinc and ASD diagnosis at different times before and after birth. For timepoints outside the yellow box, there is no relationship between zinc levels and autism (because cases and controls show no difference in zinc levels), but for times within the yellow box, the zinc levels in cases drop below those of healthy controls.

Overall, these results showed that children with ASD had lower zinc levels than their sibling during that three-month phase of life (note that the comparison is between that same time period relative to each child's birth; this is not a comparison between specific dates on the calendar). But once the children were more than one month old, we no longer see this difference between them. In this study, we uncovered what is called a "critical window of

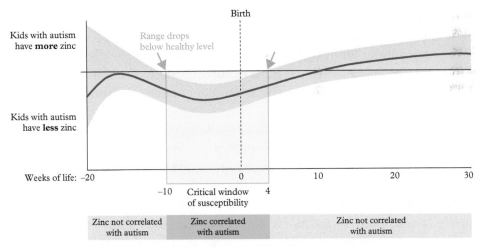

Figure 2.5 Comparison of zinc levels in teeth between autism-affected twins and their control sibling at specific developmental ages from 20 weeks before birth (part of the second and third trimesters) to 30 weeks after birth. Children with ASD had lower zinc levels in their teeth during a specific period extending from 10 weeks before birth to four weeks after birth (the yellow area). This developmental period is considered a critical window of susceptibility because it is only during this time that zinc is correlated with autism.

susceptibility" for the link between zinc uptake and autism risk—we call it so because this is a "window" in time. If we had measured zinc levels outside this window of time (for example, when the children were six months old), we would not have found that zinc levels are associated with autism diagnosis.

That was an exciting finding for us. The link between zinc and autism had been proposed before but never studied directly by using a fetal biomarker. The paper was published in a top-tier journal and was well received by our scientific peers. The implications were twofold; first, for ASD, we had identified that it is not just what the child is exposed to but also the developmental timing of the exposure that is critical to the emergence of disease. More generally, though, and returning to the themes that were introduced this chapter, our results emphasized that traditional endogenous (the nature) versus exogenous (the nurture) perspectives can never be sufficient to explain health.

The latter point might seem contradictory, given that our findings seem to strongly support an environmental contribution to the etiology of ASD. This is certainly true, but our findings also emphasize the critical role of *biological time* in the role of environmental health. Certainly, differences in zinc levels were related to ASD, but the lower levels in cases were only relevant if they occurred in the late third trimester and around birth—they were not as relevant in the second trimester, or in later childhood. As well, more generally, these findings question the premise of these strict structural dichotomies between endogenous and exogenous factors; the "exogenous" factor that is determining the child's development is occurring before the child is even born. Though not genetic, it is impossible to ignore that this "environmental" exposure is transferred in utero.

The last, and perhaps most difficult, conclusion we drew from this study was ultimately the genesis of the ideas we've come to call Environmental Biodynamics. We had set out, here, to capture the temporal dynamics underlying essential and nonessential elements; to characterize how environmental homeostasis is maintained or perturbed throughout development, and ultimately shapes human health. However, we had fallen short of that goal. In reality, we were still viewing our data through the lens of a structural perspective; we were repeating that structural analysis multiple times using our week-by-week profile of elemental uptake from the tooth biomarkers. Because of this, our analysis and interpretation were intrinsically limited to questions of organized simplicity, or disorganized complexity; that is, simple relationships between one system (the chemical exposure) and another (the developmental trajectory to ASD). We had ignored completely the emergence of *organized complexity* in elemental homeostasis and the role this might play in disease.

This was fortunately not the end of this particular journey, and in subsequent chapters we will outline the lessons we learned that ultimately led us to develop Environmental Biodynamics, which places a functional perspective at its core. As in earlier examples in real and hypothetical data, the focus in this pursuit was not to depict some static "level" and its association with our health—rather, we characterize the organization of a system over time. As studies by Scales and other colleagues have shown, this at times takes the form of analyzing biological cycles and rhythms, as in zinc homeostasis. At other times we focus instead on the formation of transient or persistent homeostatic states, or the timing and/or frequency of transitions between states. Environmental Biodynamics is ultimately the exploration of these and other dynamics that govern our homeostatic environmental equilibria, and the role of these processes in human health.

Chapter 2 Summary

Environmental medicine and related fields, including environmental epidemiology and toxicology, have developed from a structural perspective that assigns a static, anatomical "thingness" to our physiology and our environment. This viewpoint arises from a reductionist school of thought and foundational biomedical discoveries such as the discovery that human organs are made up of cells organized as tissues or that our DNA is the source "code" for the building blocks of life. As a consequence of these discoveries and their perceived importance, medical sciences have organized the study of the human body into the study of component parts. For example, so many of the textbooks we use in our medical training tend to adopt a reductionistic approach that implies a privileged role to lower levels of organization, from organs to tissues to cells to molecules, in our understanding of our health.

Attempts to incorporate *time* into existing structural perspectives have often taken the form of multiple structural analyses laced together as a circuit operating in a series of connections. Such approaches, including those under the umbrellas of "critical windows of susceptibility," "developmental origins of health and disease," and many other related paradigms, ignore core aspects of our physiology—that we and our environment are temporally dynamic processes. We, the authors, are also guilty of this, having spent much of our careers interpreting the interaction of our physiology and our environment through this lens of "thingness," and only through trial and error have we come to the realization that we cannot take the leap to a functional interpretation by simply studying more and more objects at finer spatial resolution. To overcome this, we have developed Environmental Biodynamics, a functional perspective that rejects this reductionist view of human physiology and the human environment. In stark contrast to the prevalent structural paradigms, this approach places temporal dynamics at its core. In the coming chapters we will provide the conceptual foundations and real-life examples for how Environmental Biodynamics can be operationalized.

References

1. Bai, D., et al. (2019). Association of genetic and environmental factors with autism in a 5-country cohort. *JAMA Psychiatry 76*(10), 1035–1043, doi:10.1001/jamapsychiatry.2019.1411.
2. National Human Genome Research Institute. *Genetic disorders,* https://www.genome.gov/For-Patients-and-Families/Genetic-Disorders.
3. Rappaport, S. M. (2016). Genetic factors are not the major causes of chronic diseases. *PLoS One* 11, e0154387, doi:10.1371/journal.pone.0154387.
4. Grabrucker, A. M. (2012). Environmental factors in autism. *Frontiers in Psychiatry 3,* 118.
5. Rossignol, D. A., Genuis, S. J., & Frye, R. E. (2014). Environmental toxicants and autism spectrum disorders: a systematic review. *Translational Psychiatry 4,* e360.
6. Bölte, S., Girdler, S., & Marschik, P. B. (2019). The contribution of environmental exposure to the etiology of autism spectrum disorder. *Cellular and Molecular Life Sciences 76*(7), 1275–1297.
7. Arora, M., et al. (2017). Fetal and postnatal metal dysregulation in autism. *Nature Communications* 8, 15493, doi:10.1038/ncomms15493.
8. Scales, W. E., Vander, A. J., Brown, M. B., & Kluger, M. J. (1988). Human circadian rhythms in temperature, trace metals, and blood variables. *Journal of Applied Physiology* 65, 1840–1846.

3

The Shape of Change

Complexity, Organization, and Chaos

Complexity and Organization

The first central principal of Environmental Biodynamics posits the seemingly counterintuitive notion that complex systems cannot interact directly or exist in isolation (we have called this axiom the biodynamic interface conjecture).[1] This premise has vast implications for the scientific exploration of "complex systems," which are, by definition, systems that comprise multiple subsystems. An organism is itself a complex system, being composed of systems at multiple levels of organization, from the molecular to the cellular to the level of the organs. The environment it exists in, too, is a complex system, comprising physical, chemical, biological, and social subsystems interacting on multiple spatiotemporal scales. So why can't complex systems interact directly? We eat and drink from, breathe in, and touch our environment constantly—so if we are complex systems, and the environment is a complex system, how is that these systems are not interacting *directly*?

Two essential but often overlooked truths underlie this separation. The first, which we might consider a temporal constraint, relates to the nature of how complex systems come to interact. Through the lens of a strict structural dichotomy that would divide the world into the internal (e.g., human physiology) and the external (e.g., our environment), the direct action of one distinct system upon another separate system might appear reasonable. But when the timing of this interaction is considered (When did it begin? Was there ever a moment when the biological system was not acted upon by the environment?), this separation becomes intractable. Across the vast expanse

Environmental Biodynamics. Manish Arora and Paul Curtin with Austen Curtin, Christine Austin, and Alessandro Giuliani, Oxford University Press. © Oxford University Press 2022. DOI: 10.1093/oso/9780197582947.003.0003

of time, any one moment of action of one system on another is just a drop in an ocean of prior causes. We cannot say that any one action of one system on the other drives a given outcome; rather, it is the culmination of many interactions acting in both directions. One cannot assume a specific timepoint as the beginning of an interaction. This is represented in Figure 3.1, where we might visualize the interaction of one system (A) on another system (B) but are unable to see, or are merely ignoring, the almost infinite prior interactions that culminated in this moment (the unseen interactions are in gray). In reality, there are cases when it is impossible to observe the origin point of the interaction between systems. For example, we cannot pinpoint the first position a planet occupied in its orbit around its sun. Nor does it make sense to ask whether the sun exerted its gravity on the earth first or if it was the converse. The gravitational pull of both bodies is acting in both directions *simultaneously*. Of practical relevance is the fact that this information is also not needed to fully characterize the trajectory of the planet or its interaction with its sun or other planets in the solar system. In simpler terms, Environmental

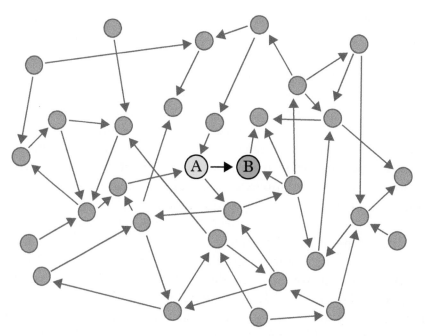

Figure 3.1 The assumption of *direct* action of a system, A, on another, B, ignores that there are a multitude of prior interactions (shown in gray) that have culminated in that spatiotemporal moment.

Biodynamics and the biodynamic interface conjecture that is at the core of this field adopt a circular bidirectional form of causality that treats the time dimension differently than it is under some current approaches that treat temporal dynamics as linear nonrecurring simple systems.

The second oft-ignored reality we don't consider in environmental health ties back to the concepts introduced by Warren Weaver in his hierarchy of information theory, and the general structure of organized complexity (discussed in Chapter 1).[2] Complex systems, themselves comprising multiple *levels* of organization, involve the coordinated interaction of multiple hierarchies. Processes at the level of the cells arise from interactions at the molecular level and, similarly, physiological systems emerge from the integration of multiple cellular process. This is to say that complex systems process information that exists at multiple levels, each sensitive to different inputs, constraints, and operations. When we integrate some aspect of the environment in our physiology—food, water, air, some adverse contact with a pollutant—that input is not integrated directly in a manner akin to organized simplicity or disorganized complexity.

One person can touch the skin of another person; what one cannot do is touch the nucleus of an atom of the skin of another person. For two people to make contact, atomic and molecular interactions give rise to cells, tissues, and organs, and interactions at those levels allow for the emergence of organism-level interactions that allow for the emergence of social norms such as touching. In the same manner as we cannot cross levels and touch a proton or an electron with our fingers, not every event at a societal level can be completely measured (and certainly not adequately explained) by using molecular markers. This fact is often forgotten in environmental epidemiological studies, for example when cortisol levels are used as the primary variable to measure social stress (cortisol is a steroid hormone; its levels increase in our body during states of heightened stimulation such as exposure to a stressful event).[3,4] It is not that cortisol levels are not linked to social stress; the point here is that cortisol levels are not *directly* linked to social stress, and it is our proposition that to adequately study that link we must consider the dynamic interfaces that mediate the transfer of information between levels across which systems are organized. This is often represented in pathway diagrams, and that practice is perfectly acceptable. However, the point we are making here is different—that at each stage of integration the environmental input is processed according to the constraints specific to that level of physiological organization, and that *dynamic interfaces* will mediate the transfer of information from that level to another, which will ultimately determine how the biological system is altered by the environmental input.

Too often, through the lens of the reductionist and structural perspectives discussed in the prior chapter, these higher and lower levels of complexity are summarily dismissed as a "metabolic process." While certainly we must resolve the role of molecular processes in human–environment interactions, in practice this perspective presents two problems. First, again, the implicit focus on assigning a privileged role of lower processes in explaining higher processes is assumed without reason. But, secondly, and more profoundly, many of the factors that would be dismissed through this rationale in fact emerge through processes that are unambiguously beyond the molecular level. Socioeconomic status, for example, can have a profound impact on the nature of our environmental homeostasis, as can our exposure to social stresses and other sociobehavioral processes. The measurement of any biological feature, at any biological level, must thus be seen through the lens of multiple dynamic processes and integrated systems; it cannot be reduced to a purely molecular agency.

Environmental Biodynamics, by focusing on *time* and embracing complexity, redefines our understanding of how complex systems influence each other, particularly in how humans and our environment impact each other. This is achieved by reversing the mistakes of the structural perspective. Rather than ignore the temporal and contextual dependencies between systems, a functional perspective makes temporal dynamics the fundamental unit of analysis; and, rather than consider isolated elements of physiological and environmental systems, we focus inquiry on the operationally independent interfaces that mediate the transfer of information between them. The points we have raised in this section—that to understand how the environment and humans interact we must consider organization in terms of time and levels of complexity—are in fact two sides of the same coin, because an interface, through the lens of Environmental Biodynamics, is the temporal dynamics that emerge from the integration of distinct systems. And these lead to a profound realization—that it is the dynamics of the interface, rather than the discrete action of either system, where the complexity that determines environmental health emerges. In this chapter, we will journey from these theoretical foundations, to focusing on principles and methods that help us quantify the interfaces we have referred to, and finally to actual health data where examining the interface gives us insight that would otherwise be missed by a purely structural approach.

The Essentiality of Biodynamic Interfaces

From the proposition that interdependent systems cannot exist in isolation comes the implication that they must at some point be integrated, and we might call this process of integration an *interface*. An interface emerges wherever the measurement of one system's state intrinsically includes inputs from another system. In measuring heart rate, for example, one can expect to capture aspects of cardiovascular health; we might notice, for example, irregularities in the cardiac rhythm that are indicative of an unhealthy heart. But at the same time our cardiovascular system serves as a common interface for a multitude of other physiological systems; excitement, anxiety, or arousal of the nervous system will also alter or disrupt the cardiac rhythm. Though the heart produces the rhythm, the physical organ itself is not the interface where the integration of these systems exists; rather, it is in the functional dynamics of the heart under varying conditions. It is in the *process* of the heart, not the structure of the heart. For that reason, tests of cardiovascular health include function, and are routinely conducted under controlled circumstances and under varying conditions of stress, in order to control for and isolate each.

This functional analysis, as is considered perfectly reasonable and standard in cardiac medicine, is the exception and not the norm in other medical fields. In environmental medicine, in our experience, the focus instead has been primarily on purely structural associations. These typically take the form of biomarker assessments, wherein concentrations of some environmental input—for example, essential nutrients or toxic chemicals—are measured in some tissue matrix such as blood or urine. These provide a momentary snapshot of how much of a given exposure is present at a given time (or might even provide a measure of cumulative exposure) but tell us nothing about the dynamics that led to and propagate the system's state.

These questions present some fundamental challenges to current standards in the design, implementation, and interpretation of environmental health studies. The first of these relates back to the temporal constraint introduced earlier in this chapter; through the static analysis of a structural perspective, we fail to consider the temporal dynamics involved in the assimilation of the environment into human physiology. Second, relating to the nature of organized complexity, a purely structural reductionist approach fails to recognize that a momentary measure of environmental inputs (the concentration of some chemical in blood, for example) does not represent the direct, isolated action of the environment upon the body; rather, it reflects a very tiny measure of the diverse host of processes linking these systems (i.e., it is a snapshot of the dynamic interface connecting us and our environment). Returning to the cardiac example, interpreting a static snapshot would be akin to measuring your heart rate throughout the day with a personal monitor, but only using a measure of heart rate at one random moment. Without consideration of your current and prior activities—resting, running, working, socializing—any given momentary measure would be meaningless. It is the same as listening to one second of a symphony, never appreciating how it began or how it ends, or all the parts in between.

The Organization of Interfaces: Determinism, Stochasticity, and Chaos

One of the most fundamental question any scientist can ask in the investigation of a given system is this: *Why is the system behaving like that?* Maybe the system is a cell in the process of mitosis, a virus propagating through a population, or an asteroid's orbit that seems curiously off course—whatever the system, the question remains the same. Environmental medicine has lost sight of this in the rigid dichotomization that arises when we adopt structuralism; we aren't concerned with the "how" or the "why" of the individual and the environment and instead seek only to describe the average or the trend. In refocusing our gaze through a functionalist lens, Environmental Biodynamics seeks to return to answering basic questions about system dynamics at the level of the biodynamic interface that connects our environment and our physiology.

Perhaps the simplest, and in many ways the most satisfying, dynamic system one might uncover is a *deterministic* system. Such a system describes some process that can be perfectly predicted through knowledge of its past; there are no random processes in its organization, and we need only know the equations that describe the system and input the relevant parameters to predict everything the system will ever do. A purely hypothetical example would be an idealized pendulum ("idealized" because it does not slow down due to friction or air resistance), which can be graphed as a sinusoidal wave function; given knowledge of its amplitude and phase angle at a given point, one can predict exactly its amplitude and phase angle at any other point forward or backward in time. Of course, perfectly deterministic systems don't usually exist in the real world for a variety of reasons, including random noise or the intervention of other processes, but many systems—planetary orbits and trajectories, for examples—are close enough that deterministic calculations yield accurate predictions for some aspects of their behavior.

The exploration of algorithms and laws underlying the world around us has been at the root of many of our greatest scientific advances and technologies; but, at a fundamental level, our reality is not, and never will be, a purely deterministic system. Many systems are better described as *stochastic*, which in the simplest sense is interpreted as having some randomly determined process. Consider molecules of air trapped in a balloon; the trajectory of any one molecule becomes incalculable as it is inevitably driven by countless collisions with other molecules, themselves subject to their own collisions. The botanist Robert Brown characterized a similar process, now known as Brownian motion, in the movement of particles suspended in water. Though stochastic processes cannot be described or predicted deterministically, because of this random unpredictability, they may still be characterized at the level of population dynamics. Because of this reason, the average behavior of molecules trapped in a balloon can be characterized as long as we study enough of them—for example, as the air in the balloon gets hotter the molecules would move more rapidly and the number of collisions would increase. Recall that in Chapter 1, we had discussed Weaver's example of how insurance companies cannot predict accurately when one person was going to die, but they have predictive models on the average behavior of different types of people to know the life expectancy of their clients.

Unfortunately, in most medical sciences, including environmental medicine, it is assumed that all systems are either deterministic or stochastic (either predictable or random). But there exists a third type—a *chaotic* system. A chaotic system exhibits some tendencies that appear superficially similar to aspects of determinism and stochasticity but are also distinct. Unlike stochastic systems, chaotic systems can be described through a system of differential equations just as a deterministic system can. However, unlike a deterministic process, the chaotic system exhibits tremendous sensitivity to initial conditions, such that even the slightest change in a system parameter yields completely different outputs. This phenomenon was extensively characterized by Edward Lorenz, a pioneer of chaos theory, in his exploration of thermodynamic equations underlying atmospheric weather conditions that exhibit chaotic properties.[5-7] His work became associated with the so-called butterfly effect, whereby even the tiniest of changes in starting could accumulate to yield vast differences in the ultimate trajectory of the system. It is often described with a hypothetical example that the change in air pressure from the flap of a butterfly's wings would influence weather patterns at faraway places. This is just one example of the practical reality that chaotic systems are incredibly difficult to predict.

These broad characterizations are models through which we understand the organization of a given system, but we must remember that when modeling an interface between two or more highly dynamic processes, like our environment and our physiology, we do not expect a "pure" manifestation of either deterministic, stochastic, or chaotic behavior. Rather, we expect, and have ourselves observed, that biodynamic interfaces integrate processes that can be readily described from all of these perspectives. The challenge then is in developing methods to characterize this dynamic complexity, and in leveraging such tools to study human health and disease.

Attractor Reconstruction: The Shape of Change

Abstract perspectives on determinism, stochasticity, and chaos provide a meaningful framework to understand the systems of the world around us— we can observe the (mostly) deterministic orbits of the celestial bodies, see the stochastic motion of pepper flakes in our soup, and experience chaos firsthand when meteorologists forecast weather. But Environmental Biodynamics does not emphasize these perspectives because of their philosophical or epistemological value; rather, these phenomena that are woven into the very fabric of our universe can be leveraged to describe, explain, and predict the organization of interfaces between ourselves and the environment. The foremost tool in solving this challenge is in the concept of the attractor, and the methods of phenomenological attractor reconstruction.

The attractor is an elusive but ubiquitous concept in the fields of dynamical systems and chaos theory. In the simplest sense, it refers to the set of points toward which a system ultimately converges.[8,9] This simple definition belies a certain implicit complexity (and beauty, which we will show later), as the "points toward which a system converges" are determined ultimately by the initial parameters of the system, the governing equations that determine its progression, and the noise present in that process from intrinsic or extrinsic forces. In Figure 3.2 we present an example system to visualize this. In panel A, we show a simple pendulum in a hypothetically idealized context (lacking

Box 3.1 On the Sequential and Synchronous Nature of Time

In Box 2.2 in Chapter 2, we had discussed the entanglement of time with change. Here, let us consider two properties of time as they relate to human biology—time is both sequential and synchronous. The ancient Greeks had two different words for the sequential and synchronous properties of time—*chronos* (sequential) time follows an ordered procession of events, but *kairos* (synchronous) time relates to how the significance of a given event depends on its interrelationship with other events. The interdependence of sequential and synchronous aspects of time is evident at all scales of organization in the world around us.

Consider, for example, an unset clock. With the introduction of VCR and DVD players, prior to the use of networked synchronization, the ubiquitous blinking light of the unset VCR/DVD player clock at "12:00" all day long was common in many households. Here was a device perfectly attuned to measure the procession of time, but without an external cue—a *zeitgeber* (German for "time giver," the stimulus a clock is set to)—the clock's time-keeping capacity is rendered meaningless. Although its mechanism to measure intervals of time might be precise, the clock can be rendered thoroughly inaccurate by failing to synchronize it with a reference time (such as Greenwich Mean Time plus or minus your time zone difference). Imagine that you are tired of the unceasing blinking of "12:00" but not bothered enough to set it properly, so one evening, in frustration, you simply press the "set" button at some random time, thereby programing the device to start marking time beginning at 12:00. From that point forward, the clock would keep an accurate measure of the sequential procession of time, but that time would be irrelevant and inaccurate to the local time because of its lack of synchronization to other events and processes related to the clock.

Similarly, in biological systems, both sequential and synchronous temporal processes are critical. From the moment of conception, embryos undergo successive stages of cellular division, proliferation, and differentiation, with each stage of an organ's development dependent on preceding events within that specific organ as well as on concurrent changes in other developing organs. Much research has been done to characterize these processes in a strictly structural sense; the questions that have been asked are akin to asking how different components of a clock connect to each other. Environmental Biodynamics, however, asks deeper questions and seeks to determine how to characterize a biological system in sequential and synchronous *functional* terms; in other words, how different clocks across vastly different scales work in unison.

---

friction, wind resistance, and other forces that would throw it off course). This is a classical example of a purely deterministic process, as its motion can be described entirely as a function of its mass, the length of the pendulum shaft, and the angle of the starting position. If we track its velocity over time,

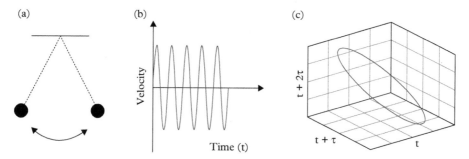

Figure 3.2 Example of a deterministic system. Panel A shows an idealized pendulum that does not slow down once set into motion. The side-to-side motion of this pendulum can be plotted as a sine wave (panel B) but can also be visualized as an orbit by plotting the velocity of the pendulum against temporally-lagged dimensions (tau). The elliptical orbit of the pendulum shown in panel C is termed the "limit cycle attractor."

as in panel B, we see the formation of a purely sinusoidal process as one would expect from such a deterministic system—that is, the side-to-side motion of the pendulum that we see can be plotted as a line that moves up and down in a regular pattern as a function of time. In panel C we show the attractor underlying this system, which in many ways is its orbit; to be more technically specific, we show that this system is governed by what is called a limit-cycle attractor.

The limit cycle attractor, so called because its closed-form trajectory captures every possible state of the system, allows us to assess the organization of a given system.[10,11] The attractor is reconstructed through the application of Takens delay-embedding,[12,13] whereby the original observations of a given system—here, the velocity of the pendulum measured over time (marked t in panel C)—is plotted against a time-lagged vector of observations (in panel C, t represents the original series of velocity measures, while t + tau and t + 2tau reflect vectors of t lagged by interval tau). In essence, the system is embedded in itself to characterize its movement through time. The attractor underlying this system emerged as an elliptical orbit because the pendulum's movement was perfectly cyclical. The absence of noise and the perfect predictability of the system confirms for us that this is a deterministic system.

The reconstruction of the attractor thus provides an answer to the question that we asked at the beginning of our exploration of system dynamics: *Why is this system behaving like that?* In the case of the pendulum, it is swinging back and forth because the system is "stuck" in a limit cycle—the attractor that organizes the system is a closed-form loop. This allows for a high-level summary of the system but also provides a means for practical measurements of the system's dynamics. We can now, for example, measure the system in terms of its dynamical organization: What is the diameter of this attractor? How long does it take to complete one whole loop on its orbit? And how stable is its trajectory? These are examples of the functional measures we can use to characterize dynamic interfaces that integrate physiological and environmental systems—measures of organized complexity *in time*, which capture the "how" and the "why" of our physiology.

We can also extend these methods to different types of systems. In Figure 3.3 we introduce a modified system—here, a double pendulum. This system is identical to the previous pendulum, but now a second pendulum shaft and a mass (the sphere at the end) have been attached to the first pendulum. We see a dramatic shift in the underlying system's trajectory (shown on the right). Rather than merely alter some parameters of the system (its velocity, for example), the addition of a second pendulum caused a fundamental shift in the nature of the system's dynamics—a butterfly effect, so to speak. While a single pendulum is a deterministic system, when we examine a double pendulum

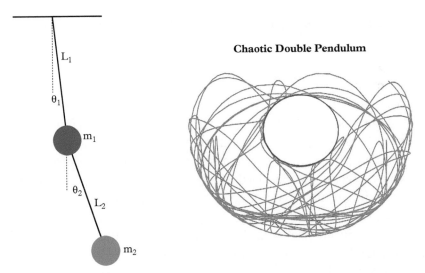

Figure 3.3 On the left is a double pendulum comprising two pendulums with length (L) and mass (m). Angles θ_1 and θ_2 denote the initial system parameters. The path when only a single pendulum is active is shown by the blue circle. The addition of the second ball causes the regular pendulum (a deterministic system) to become chaotic. A trace of the path taken by the second ball in a double pendulum is shown in red.

the system becomes chaotic and unpredictable. You will notice the stark contrast between the path of the single pendulum, shown as the blue circle, with the path taken by the double pendulum, shown by the red line.

The additional ball turned a perfectly deterministic and predictable system, and consequently a fundamentally timeless system (given that it is bounded by a perpetual limit cycle), into a far more complex dynamic system that changes continuously in a manner that is difficult to predict. As an interesting aside, this complex and exotic behavior of a double pendulum signifies an age-old problem in dynamic systems theory, known as the three-body problem (we discuss this further in Chapter 4).

Overall, attractor reconstruction provides an essential insight into the nature of the system we observe; does it change according to a deterministic regime, or is it subject to chaos or to random noise? More importantly, it provides a concrete basis for a functional analysis of system dynamics. A variety of other methods will also be explored throughout this book to achieve this end, focusing on the measurement of dynamics in the context of determinism, periodicity, complexity, and stability, all of which will provide quantitative measures of the biodynamic interface.

Incorporating Biodynamics and the Shape of Change into Precision Medicine

How do we incorporate time and biodynamic interfaces in the way we practice environmental medicine? In the previous chapter we illustrated how reductionist perspectives focus on the characterization of distributions of static measurements at the level of a population. In that view the measures of interest are descriptive statistics such as the mean or the median, and measures of variability such as the standard deviation or the confidence interval. That approach is inherently structural, or anatomical; the environmental input we measure is interpreted as a static "level," and we seek to understand how the level of the input relates to the distribution of some health outcome. In Environmental Biodynamics we propose a functional alternative and, of the several methods at its core, attractor reconstruction in an important one that we have outlined in the preceding section.

Just as, to a structuralist, the population distribution provides a means of characterizing a static measurement (see Chapter 2), in a functional perspective the form of the underlying attractor system provides the means of

Box 3.2 Artistic Aside

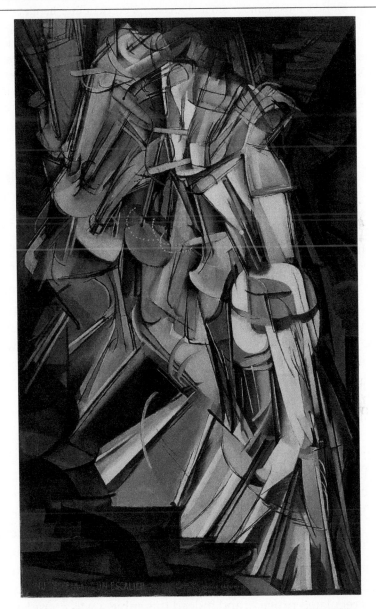

You might wonder how this painting by Marcel Duchamp—*Nu descendant un escalier n°
2* (Nude Descending a Staircase, No. 2)—is relevant to our discussion on attractors. At
their core, this painting and an attractor both show how a system evolves in time. This
painting is different to other masterpieces; for example, Leonardo da Vinci's *Mona Lisa*

doesn't show her facial expression before or after she has finished posing with what is perhaps the world's most famous smile. Duchamp, on the other hand, has managed something unique by conveying the position of the system he was studying—the subject depicted in the painting—at different locations in her trajectory down the staircase.

The limit-cycle attractor does the same thing for the pendulum by showing us the different locations it occupies in its orbit, and later in this chapter, we present an attractor showing the temporal path of how our body metabolizes the essential element copper for a period of almost 10 years. Like Duchamp's masterpiece, that attractor will also show, in a single graphic, a system's trajectory over time.

characterizing the *shape of change* at the level of the individual. This provides, in itself, useful insights into the organization of a given system as well as serving as the basis for subsequent measurements. Consider the following two examples to illustrate these points.

In our first example, we introduce data generously provided through the PhysioNet resource maintained by the Massachusetts Institute of Technology (MIT).[14] In keeping with our emphasis on physiological approaches, we accessed MIT's PhysioNet archive to analyze electrocardiograms (ECGs) collected under similar conditions from four subjects with varying degrees of cardiac health. In the top panel of Figure 3.4, we show the raw data collected from each subject. For our purposes, a brief (four-second) snippet of the ECG is shown. In the bottom panels we show the attractors reconstructed from each signal, derived identically to the procedure used in the analysis of the pendulum in the prior section.

In the left-most subject, we see the emergence of a highly orderly system, very much reminiscent of the limit-cycle observed in the single pendulum, though with additional complexity and the presence of noise, as is inevitable in biological systems. This orderly system progresses through a tight loop (at lower left) and then a broad orbital swing and return (longer loop to right and top), reflective of the underlying ECG dynamics, which include both low-level baseline fluctuations (corresponding to atrial depolarization and ventricular repolarization) and the high peak of the pulsing ventricular depolarization. The persistent regularity and stability of this system is indicative of a tightly regulated process, and indeed this subject was considered to be in perfectly good cardiac health.

The other recordings were taken from subjects with clinical cardiac abnormalities, and these are apparent in the distorted attractors that emerge from

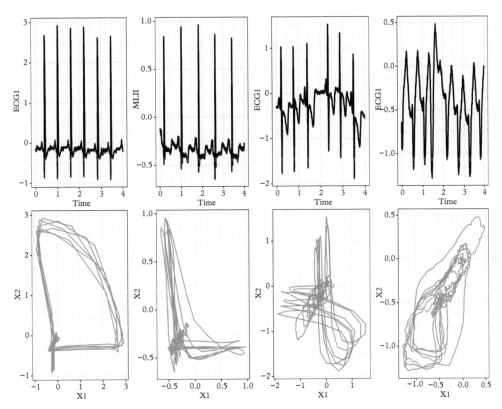

Figure 3.4 Attractor reconstruction from ECGs collected in standardized conditions. Top panels show raw data, while bottom panels show underlying attractor systems. From left to right, data were collected from subjects who were healthy or diagnosed with arrhythmia, atrial fibrillation, or malignant ventricular arrhythmia, respectively.

their cardiac dynamics. In the middle-left panel, we show at top the raw ECG recorded in a subject with cardiac arrhythmia. To the untrained eye the raw ECG does not immediately present a stark contrast with the healthy signal, but the disorganization of the underlying attractor system is glaring. In the middle-right and right-most panels these patterns are further exacerbated in patients with atrial fibrillation (middle-right) and malignant ventricular arrhythmia. These patterns are certainly not stochastic, as there remains a clear orbital trajectory in the procession of the signal, but the near-deterministic precision of the healthy heart has been displaced by an unstable process.

These examples emphasize the utility of attractor reconstruction and functional, physiological analyses in biomedical science. Rather than analyze measures of intensity or simple measures of change, such as rate, the attractor allows us to analyze the nature of the underlying *system*, and to return to the fundamental questions we began with: *Why is the system behaving this way?* In the case of the healthy individual, cardiac dynamics are organized in a stable orbital system reminiscent of a limit cycle, and we can consequently expect the system to maintain this stable trajectory in time. In these cases of cardiac disease, we see this stability successively degenerated with increasing severity; while arrhythmia appears governed by an unstable but recognizable limit cycle, atrial defibrillation and ventricular arrhythmia involve the emergence of increasingly dysregulated dynamics.

Critically, the utility of this approach is not limited to the analysis of complex systems, or dependent on high-resolution temporal sampling; in fact, all that is needed are successive measures of a system of interest. To emphasize this in a more familiar context, we introduce data collected from a very personal source: the weight-loss recordings of one of the authors. Like many people, this particular author had gained some weight during the seasonal holidays; and, with some spousal encouragement, ultimately decided it was time to "shed some pounds." To achieve this, he commenced a diet-based weight-loss program for three months, with morning weigh-ins recorded daily under standardized conditions to track his progress.

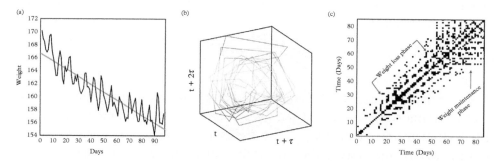

Figure 3.5 Graphic depictions of Author A's weight loss. Additional clinically meaningful information is revealed as we move from a purely structural analysis (shown in panel A) to examining the biodynamic interface mediating the impact of diet modification on weight loss (panels B and C). In panel B, we have constructed an attractor that reveals an orbital trajectory to this weight-loss pattern. And in panel C, we analyze the data from the attractor to show when Author A departs from the linear trend and enters a period of weight maintenance; in the recurrence plot, this is apparent as an expansion of recurrence plots away from the diagonal line, indicating a persistently revisited state (top right corner).

The raw data from morning weigh-ins are shown in Figure 3.5, panel A. From a broad perspective, this illustrates some simple good news: The author clearly succeeded, to some extent, in reducing his bodyweight. But a closer examination reveals there are underlying patterns in this trajectory that aren't entirely consistent with diligence and good behavior. First, in a broad sense, the weight loss seems to happen primarily during the start of the dietary period; there is a period toward the end of this diet where weight loss seems to level off. Second, even on days when bodyweight was declining, there appear to be some strange oscillations, almost as if there was a cycle underlying this author's weight, upon which the weight loss was superimposed. In fact, these cycles corresponded to some predictable lapses in the author's dietary protocols—while he diligently regulated caloric intake during the work week, all bets were off on the weekends. This delinquency yielded a pattern of repetitive weight loss and gain.

Superimposed on these data, we illustrate a simple linear fit (blue line) that exemplifies the traditional structural perspective on these patterns. In this context the important measure is the global trend, which is captured in the slope of the linear fit. Certainly, this tells us some important things about this pattern of change—in general, that the overall trend was negative, consistent with weight loss over time, and more specifically it tells us, on average, what the *rate* of loss was per day. These measures are useful, but they tell us nothing about the dynamic *interface* between this author's diet, his activities, and the homeostatic processes involved in the maintenance of his weight.

The functional perspective of Environmental Biodynamics is as applicable to these data as it was to pendulums and cardiac dynamics. In Figure 3.4, panel B, we show the attractor underlying this author's weight-loss trajectory. This reveals a system that oscillates in a steady manner, but over time the focal point of this orbital trajectory seems to shift. Indeed, this tracks with what is observed in the raw data—a rhythm superimposed on a declining trend. As well, we see that over time the diameter of these orbits seems to decline, becoming ultimately tighter. The flattening of the trend toward the lower right of the graph in panel A and the tightening of the orbit in panel B reflect reaching the limit of diet-related weight loss; that is, in order to continue to lose weight, one would have to introduce another strategy, perhaps making a different dietary modification or adding exercise.

Unlike prior reconstructions we have shown, we will here extend our analysis further to a quantitative perspective on the attractor dynamics underlying this system. For this we utilize a method called recurrence quantification analysis (RQA), which, generally speaking, does exactly what you would expect from its name. That is, with RQA we analyze the *timing* of repetitions within a system—of recurrences—in order to measure properties such as the prevalence, duration, and complexity of cyclical properties in a given attractor system. This method yields a graphical representation, called a recurrence plot, which we show in Figure 3.4C (additional details of RQA are given in the appendix).

The recurrence plot offers a graphical depiction of the timing of recurrences in a given system. Both X- and Y-axes represent timing within a given system; one can trace along the X-axis to a given timepoint—here, say day 20—then move up along the Y-axis. The appearance of black dots represents a moment where the system re-enters a state it was in at a given time-point—a black dot at 20 on the X-axis and 30 on the Y-axis means that at 30 days, the system re-entered the state it was in at 20 days. When systems engage in periodic behavior, this construction inevitably forces the emergence of black diagonal lines, as the points adjacent to each other will also recur sequentially. This allows a quick visual assessment of periodic processes and is also easily quantified; we can, for example, use this tool to measure orbital durations. In other words, whereas attractor reconstruction provides a high-level visualization of system dynamics, RQA provides a means to *quantify* and measure the dynamics of the attractor.

In this context, with respect to Figure 3.5, the recurrence analysis of the weight-loss attractor reveals two general patterns. First, during the period of weight loss, we see diagonal lines emerging close to the main diagonal. These are indicative of the weekly weight-loss cycles; they remain close to the diagonal because the system does not return to states it was in near the beginning of the period (due to the weight loss). Toward the end of this period, we see the emergence of a new dynamic evident in the top right corner, where we see the diagonal structure suddenly expand to form a wider square. This indicates that the system has reached a stable plateau.

Both structural and functional perspectives thus each provided some insight as to the overall weight-loss trajectory, but the functional analysis allowed additional information into the nature of the system and how it was integrating dietary and lifestyle changes. Far from a simple linear trend, in fact this system included multiple physiologically relevant dynamics, including a weekly oscillation that persisted through weight loss, and an overall homeostatic shift from a weight-loss regimen to a weight-maintenance regimen.

Taken together, how can the functional analytical perspectives emphasized in Environmental Biodynamics be leveraged to advance personalized medicine? In contrast to the population-based focus of reductionism and structuralism, the focus on individualized physiology in the functional approach provides insights into the fundamental organization of a given biological system. In current practice it is common to hear one's health summarized as a list of measures, such as "your LDL cholesterol increased by 10 mg/dL" or "you lost five pounds in the last six months." But from the perspective of Environmental Biodynamics, we should instead be focusing on the organization of homeostatic processes, whether at the level of lipid metabolism or weight loss. We should be asking, instead, how stable is the orbit of your cholesterol levels (here, by "orbit" we are referring to the trajectory of the attractor) or the dynamics of *complexity* in your nutrient profiles. Whereas traditional medical models treat disease after symptoms become obvious, approaches that consider biodynamic interfaces can help create diagnostic tools to apply before symptoms arise by focusing on the organization of underlying systems and detecting divergences from healthy orbits.

Environmental Biodynamics and Environmental Medicine (Case Studies)

In the previous section we introduced the study of organized complexity using attractor reconstruction in physiological systems. Similar approaches can be applied to study environmental systems, but ultimately the focus of Environmental Biodynamics is explicitly on the interfaces that connect environmental and physiological systems.

To achieve this, we return to the biomarker technology outlined in Chapter 2, which enabled our initial explorations of time-varying dynamics. This approach leveraged the unique biology of tooth development to generate retrospective temporal biomarkers that allowed us to reconstruct the history of chemical exposures in a child from the second trimester of pregnancy through the first year of life (in essence, teeth have growth rings like trees, and we can measure different chemicals along those growth rings to generate a timeline of exposure). We focused our analysis on essential elements, such as zinc, copper, and manganese, as these are necessary for healthy development. As well we analyzed toxic metals in order to compare how these were processed relative to essential nutrients. Whereas the prior study (described in Chapter 2) employed an essentially structural approach, focusing solely on elemental concentrations, here we focused on revealing the organized complexity of the biodynamic interface by analyzing elemental attractor systems.

Our initial efforts focused on a purely exploratory analysis of elemental homeostasis. This was, at the time, an entirely novel and unproven approach, and we were not entirely certain what we would find. Although the prior studies we have discussed, such as the findings of Wendy Scales's group (see Chapter 2), had observed cycles in elemental homeostasis, those studies had focused entirely on circadian rhythms over the course of just a few days. Our measurements, in contrast, encompassed more than a year of biological development, and we were not limiting ourselves to only deterministic systems (such as a cyclical pattern) but also wanted to observe underlying stochastic and chaotic patterns.

To ensure the robust generalizability of our results, we employed a dual cohort design in our initial exploratory study. In this approach we focused our initial assessments on one cohort of healthy children, recruited in Sweden, with whom we could establish an initial characterization of system dynamics. Our plan was then to attempt generalizing these findings to an entirely different cohort far across the world in the United States. If we could show these patterns were consistent in such different populations, it would support the idea that the biodynamical pattern is an integral part of normal human physiology.

Contrary to our initial concerns that these systems might lack dynamic complexity, we found that we had underestimated the sophisticated organization underlying elemental assimilation into our bodies. In Figure 3.6 we show two example traces derived from analyses of children's teeth; on the left, the time-varying magnitude of calcium, and at right, copper. In each we see two very different regimes that would subsequently become the focus of multiple investigations. In the calcium, we see a regular, sinusoidal oscillation reminiscent of the pendulum, or even the heart; and, indeed, exploration of the underlying attractor system revealed a near-limit cycle organization in this system. In the copper, at right, we observed a different dynamic that we will later return to—rather than form a persistent limit cycle, we see the emergence of two discrete attractor states. It seemed as if copper was "jumping" from one attractor to another throughout development. Here, now, we were able to answer that most important, but elusive, of questions—*What is the orbit of my calcium metabolism (or, for that matter, my copper level, my blood pressure, heart rate, weight loss, cholesterol level, or any other physiological feature)?*

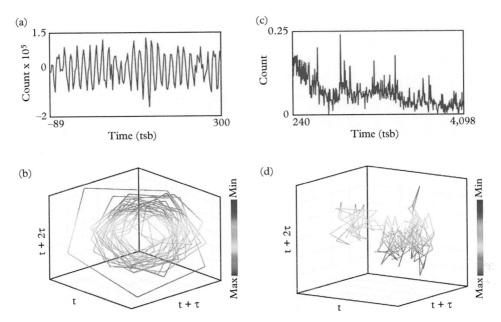

Figure 3.6 A functional analysis of the biodynamics underlying assimilation of calcium (panels A, B) and copper (panels C, D) reveals stark differences in the attractor profiles of both essential elements. Calcium metabolism appears to be organized as a limit cycle attractor (similar to a pendulum), whereas copper appears to follow a bistable attractor, "jumping" from one stable state to another during its metabolic trajectory. In panels A and C, element concentrations are measured as counts (concentration) and developmental time is indicated as time since birth (tsb) in days. In panels B and D, t represents the original series of velocity measures, while t + tau and t + 2tau reflect vectors of t lagged by interval tau.

While attractor reconstruction provided qualitative insights into the organization of these systems, we relied on RQA, which we had previously applied in the weight-loss example, to quantify and measure cyclical attractor dynamics. Recall that this method focuses on quantifying the cycle prevalence, duration, and complexity (or, in technical terms used by computational biologists, determinism, diagonal length, and entropy). Consistent with our focus on personalized dynamics, we measured these features in each elemental pathway, at the level of the individual (that is, in each child) and did not rely on a population average.

When we looked at data from the other nutrient elements and toxic metals, the patterns that emerged were clear and unambiguous. To illustrate how big the contrast is between the two approaches, we first show a graph with

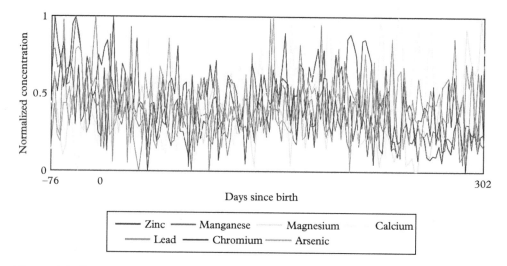

Figure 3.7 Example of an individual's elemental time series ranging from 76 days before birth to 302 days after birth. Elemental concentrations were normalized between 0 and 1. No clear pattern emerged to distinguish toxic from nutritive elements.

only the concentration of the different elements we had measured (that is, a purely structural view of our data)—this is shown in Figure 3.7. The readers will notice that it is hard to distinguish any clear difference between essential nutrients and toxic metals. However, when we explore the biodynamics of elemental assimilation, a very different, and much clearer, picture emerges (Figure 3.8). In one group of elements, including calcium, zinc, copper, manganese, and magnesium, the complexity (entropy) of cyclical attractor dynamics was persistently high. In another group of elements, including lead, chromium, and arsenic, the complexity of attractor systems was significantly diminished. This pattern perfectly coincided with 50 years of toxicological studies—we had found, in essence, that homeodynamics of essential elements exhibit robust organized complexity, while toxic or nonessential elements do not. This pattern stayed true in our replication population in the United States (Figure 3.8, bottom panel).[15]

These findings were a profound revelation for us and offered a roadmap for the practical implementation of the functional perspective that would later become Environmental Biodynamics. That is, where other studies understood the environment through an examination of static concentrations of exposure, we would apply RQA and related dynamical methods to characterize the complexity of underlying attractor systems mediating elemental

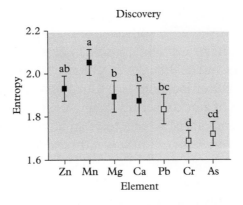

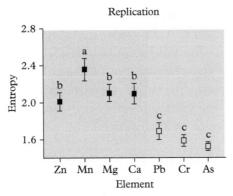

Figure 3.8 Discovery in Sweden and replication in the United States. Entropy values (a measure of a system's complexity) in nutrient (pink) and toxicant (blue) elements. Compared to data shown in Figure 3.7, essential and toxic metals are clearly distinguished. Lowercase letters indicate which elements are similar and which are different in their entropy measures; elements sharing a letter do not statistically differ.

Source: Curtin P et al. (2017). Recurrence quantification analysis to characterize cyclical components of environmental elemental exposures during fetal and postnatal development. *PLoS One* 12(11), e0187049, doi:10.1371/journal.pone.0187049.

homeostasis. The next step to achieve this was to demonstrate the importance of these processes to human health and development.

Given our initial explorations of elemental exposures in autism spectrum disorder, as described in Chapter 2, we decided to return to this study armed with the tools of a functional analysis. With this investigation, unlike the last, where we were ourselves viewing our data through a structural lens, we were also able to simultaneously expand our cohort to a discovery-replication design. Rather than focus on a single cohort of twins, drawn from the Roots of Autism Twin Study (RATSS) in Sweden, we instead recruited cohorts from all around the world. With subjects from Texas, New York, the United Kingdom, and Sweden, we were finally able to explore the interface between environmental factors and healthy development.[16]

In children from all four locations, we found some surprisingly consistent results. Three aspects of zinc dynamics (again, the reader may think of this as the orbit of zinc's metabolism) were altered in autism—the zinc cycles were shorter in time, they were less complex, and they tended to have more periods of irregularity. Even more interesting was that the disruptions of the zinc cycle were not happening in isolation; rather, the orbit of zinc was dependent on the orbit of copper. This is akin to two musicians playing together in harmony, but in the case of autism the duo was playing out of sync. Specifically, the combined zinc–copper cycles were disrupted in children with autism from all four centers in three different countries. In Figure 3.9 we show one piece of our findings—the complexity of the joint orbits of zinc and copper. You will see how children with autism have lower complexity, indicating that dynamics involved in the joint zinc–copper cycles have been compromised. Even though at the time of writing of this book we do not know all the details

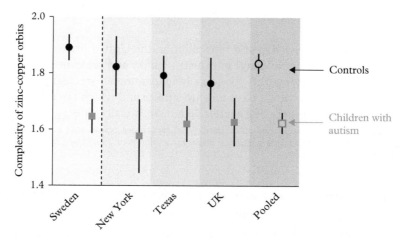

Figure 3.9 Disruption of zinc-copper orbits in autism spectrum disorder. Data show the complexity (entropy) of zinc–copper cycles (higher numbers on the Y-axis represent greater complexity). Controls (children without an autism diagnosis) show higher levels of complexity than children with the disorder.

Pooled estimates generated by combining data from all sites. Data are means ± 95% confidence intervals.

Source: Curtin P et al. (2018). Dynamical features in fetal and postnatal zinc-copper metabolic cycles predict the emergence of autism spectrum disorder. *Science Advances* 4(5), eaat1293, doi:10.1126/sciadv.aat1293.

of the molecular basis of zinc's action in autism, we did show a remarkable correlation at the level of the individual (not a population average) between dynamic descriptors of zinc fluctuations and the onset of autism. Moreover, in the Swedish participants, this result was shown in twins, which at least partially controls for any direct influence of the base genetic sequence.

These results were, from our perspective, something of a breakthrough—we had shown that elemental biodynamics was critical to healthy neurodevelopment and were dysregulated in disease. Later, in Chapter 4, we will expand on these themes to show how this approach could be extended beyond descriptive perspectives on disease to clinical utility—we will go further to the development of highly accurate predictive models, which have enormous implications for how we consider the origins of disease. The approaches outlined here are nonetheless meant to serve as just a brief introduction to the possibilities of a functional analysis; insightful, we hope, but insufficient to resolve other aspects of complexity we will inevitably encounter in biological systems, including pattern formation, state dependency, interdependence, and mutual constraints. We will explore these topics further in subsequent chapters.

Chapter 3 Summary

We opened this chapter with the first central principle of Environmental Biodynamics—that complex systems cannot interact directly, nor exist in isolation. We also introduced the corollary principle that although the interface is composed of constant change (i.e., processes), it retains a quantifiable topography—the shape of change—driven by stochastic, deterministic, or chaotic processes. The implication of this, from the perspective of environmental medicine, is that the environment and human physiology are integrated via an *interface*. An interface emerges wherever the measurement of one system's state intrinsically includes inputs from another system. And thus, to understand how the environment influences us, and vice versa, environmental medicine must adopt a functional perspective that focuses on the organization of system dynamics and complexity. This is achieved by characterizing the deterministic, stochastic, and chaotic processes that shape environmental homeostasis (which we explored here through two methods—attractor reconstruction and recurrence quantification analysis).

This paradigm shift has profound implications for the practice of environmental medicine. The functional perspective of Environmental Biodynamics implicitly focuses inquiry at the level of the individual rather than the population; as such it provides a platform for precision medicine, while at the same time offering a new scientific paradigm. We have shown the utility of this, generally, in our investigations of essential nutrients and toxic elements. More specifically, we have shown that the complexity of cyclical processes in elemental assimilation is unambiguously critical to healthy development, as we found that these features, particularly involving zinc and copper metabolism, were dysregulated in autism spectrum disorder.

More generally, the perspective of Environmental Biodynamics reflects an effort to refocus our understanding of environmental health on the nature of organized complexity. Where reductionist perspectives have entrained us to envision environmental inputs as static constants, a functional perspective views the integration of the environment as an ongoing *process* with *time* at its very core. This process is part of our inheritance as much as it is a part of our environment; it has shaped, and been shaped, through our development and plays a critical role throughout the whole of the human life.

References

1. Arora, M., Giuliani, A., & Curtin, P. (2020). Biodynamic interfaces are essential for human–environment interactions. *Bioessays* **42**, e2000017, doi:10.1002/bies.202000017.
2. Weaver, W. (1948). Science and complexity. *American Scientist* **36**, 536–544.
3. Stalder, T., et al. (2017). Stress-related and basic determinants of hair cortisol in humans: a meta-analysis. *Psychoneuroendocrinology* **77**, 261–274, https://doi.org/10.1016/j.psyneuen.2016.12.017.
4. Sapolsky, R. M., Romero, L. M., & Munck, A. U. (2000). How do glucocorticoids influence stress responses? Integrating permissive, suppressive, stimulatory, and preparative actions. *Endocrine Reviews* **21**, 55–89.
5. Lorenz, E. N. (1963). Deterministic nonperiodic flow. *Journal of the Atmospheric Sciences* **20**(2), 130–141.
6. Lorenz, E. N. (1969). Atmospheric predictability as revealed by naturally occurring analogues. *Journal of the Atmospheric Sciences* **26**(4), 636–646.
7. Gleick, J. (1987). *Chaos: Making a New Science.* Cardinal, p. 17. ISBN 978-0-434-29554-8.
8. Weisstein, E. W. Attractor. *MathWorld,* https://mathworld.wolfram.com/Attractor.html.
9. Milnor, J. (1985). On the concept of attractor. *Communications in Mathematical Physics* **99**(2), 177–195, doi:10.1007/BF01212280.

10. Roenneberg, T., Chua, E. J., Bernardo, R., & Mendoza, E. (2008). Modelling biological rhythms. *Current Biology* **18**(17), R826–R835, doi:10.1016/j.cub.2008.07.017.
11. Mackey, M., & Glass, L. (1977). Oscillation and chaos in physiological control systems. *Science* **197**(4300), 287–289, doi:10.1126/science.267326.
12. Takens, F. (1981). Detecting strange attractors in turbulence. In D. Rand & L-S. Young (Eds.), *Dynamical Systems and Turbulence, Lecture Notes in Mathematics* (Vol. 898, pp. 366–381). Springer-Verlag.
13. Abarbanel, H. (1996). *Analysis of Observed Chaotic Data.* Springer-Verlag.
14. Goldberger, A.L., et al. (2000). PhysioBank, PhysioToolkit, and PhysioNet: Components of a new research resource for complex physiologic signals. *Circulation* **101**(23), e215–e220, doi:10.1161/01.CIR.101.23.e215.
15. Curtin, P., et al. (2017). Recurrence quantification analysis to characterize cyclical components of environmental elemental exposures during fetal and postnatal development. *PloS One* **12**, e0187049, doi:10.1371/journal.pone.0187049.
16. Curtin, P., et al. (2018). Dynamical features in fetal and postnatal zinc-copper metabolic cycles predict the emergence of autism spectrum disorder. *Science Advances* **4**(5), eaat1293, doi:10.1126/sciadv.aat1293.

4

The Process of Interdependence

Temporal Dynamics of Biodynamic Interfaces

Introduction

We could define or describe any given system in this universe by any given set
of measures and find that all systems have one thing in common: *They cannot
exist in isolation.* From the simplest to the most complex, every process relies
on the integration of some input to generate some corresponding output,
mediated via an interface, which will inevitably provide inputs to other processes that may be active concurrently or at a later timepoint. The cascading
procession of interdependencies governing physical, chemical, and biological processes provides the fundamental organizational matrix of life, and is
accordingly the major focus of many emerging and frequently overlapping
scientific fields. Similarly, a key aspect of what we are proposing here is to leverage these interdependencies to understand the role of the environment in
human health or, in other words, to understand how we are connected to our
environment.

As always, in the application of Environmental Biodynamics, the fundamental unit in understanding the role of the environment in health is in
studying the temporally dynamic interface at which the environment and
human physiology influence each other. That is, rather than focus only on
the concentration or the "how much" of an environmental exposure, we seek
to understand the persistent exchange and interaction involved in environmental exposures and their assimilation. In Chapter 3, we described the concept of the *shape of change* that allows us to visualize the architecture of the
dynamics of the environment and our physiology. We also outlined a variety

Environmental Biodynamics. Manish Arora and Paul Curtin with Austen Curtin, Christine Austin, and Alessandro Giuliani, Oxford University Press. © Oxford University Press 2022. DOI: 10.1093/oso/9780197582947.003.0004

of methodologies useful in achieving this, including attractor reconstruction, recurrence analysis, and related dynamical methods (see the appendix for details). Now, in this chapter, we turn our attention to the relationships and interdependencies among these processes. In the broadest terms, here we will focus on how our physiology deals with the interplay between the myriad of environmental factors, some of which are good for our health and others, detrimental. How, for example, is the assimilation of a given nutrient enhanced by the metabolism of other nutrients or disrupted by exposure to a toxic chemical? Further, in characterizing relationships between two systems, can we measure how these are embedded in a larger system of interdependencies? The ultimate goal, thus, includes not only discrete analyses of synchronicities that tie systems together but also characterizations of systemwide organization.

Models of Interdependence

To begin to approach this problem, consider the simplest form of interdependence between two systems—a connection of two interacting processes. From the structural perspective, this immediately suggests an associative or correlational framework. This would be modeled or studied by measuring the activation of one system (let's call it A) and measuring the corresponding change in another system (let's call it B). This is, of course, perfectly reasonable—if two systems are related, then changes in one *should* relate to changes in another, and the traditional statistical approaches to characterizing these (such as linear models) are perfectly adequate in characterizing the magnitude, direction, and statistical significance of associations like this. This approach is additionally advantageous in that it can be generalized to virtually any two systems; we could measure the magnitude of some environmental exposure, such as air pollution, and link this to a corresponding change in some neurodevelopmental measure in children, such as IQ; or, we could measure changes in one physiological system, such as heart rate, and link it to changes in another, such as blood oxygenation.

The problem with this approach, however, is that it ignores the underlying dynamic interfaces that connect these systems; associations between static measures of system A and static measures of system B do nothing to inform us of *how* one system came to be dependent on the other. Two critical elements are missing in this approach, which Environmental Biodynamics seeks to integrate in our perspective on environmental medicine. The first of these is the integration of *time* in how we characterize the dependency of one system upon another; through an examination of the temporal dynamics linking two systems, we can better understand the nature of their connection. Second, we must understand the fundamental truth with which we introduced this chapter—that *no system exists in isolation.* As such, we must understand the dependency of any given system both on its own past, as previously emphasized, and on its sensitivity to perturbation from the environment.

To illustrate these principles, consider again the example of two hypothetical systems, A and B. These could be mechanisms involved in any hypothesized biological process involving interacting systems; two circuits that activate sequentially to control some motor function, for example, like the contraction of a bicep and corresponding inhibition of the triceps, but given our focus on environmental health, let's assume these are two molecules whose relative concentrations are mutually regulated. Rather than take some static measure of their output as we did previously—say, IQ to summarize some aspect of brain function, or a measure of air pollution to summarize the environment— we will instead characterize the *temporal* processes that relate one system to another, which in this example will include two simple regulatory mechanisms that we might find at every level of organization in human physiology.

The first, called *reciprocal inhibition,* allows A to exert an inhibitory control over B that is proportional to its concentration; this means that increasing concentrations of A will force a reduction in concentrations of B. Likewise, the same control is exerted by B on A. This reciprocal inhibition effectively creates a *positive feedback loop,* which generally indicates that the activation of a given process stimulates additional activation of the process. We will include an additional regulatory mechanism, called an auto-inhibitory circuit, which will cause either system to be suppressed if its concentration becomes too high. This process of feedback inhibition creates a *negative feedback loop* that ensures that concentrations of A and B remain constrained within a certain range; they cannot become "too high" because they are shut off when they go beyond a certain limit, much like a thermostat. The positive and negative feedback loops are diagrammed in the top panel of Figure 4.1.[1]

The organization of this static topological circuit, which balances the positive feedback imposed by reciprocal inhibition and the negative feedback of auto-inhibition, predicts a balanced system that we expect to give rise to almost identical concentrations of A and B—that is, we expect that it would behave like a seesaw with a small range of motion but keeping both sides in

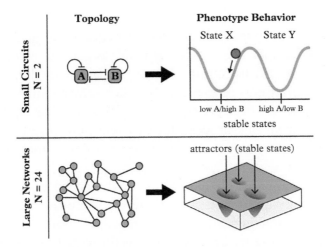

Figure 4.1 Schematic representation of a biological circuit with feedback loops and reciprocal inhibition. Process A or B, when activated, will inhibit the other until deactivated by a recurrent inhibitory process. This yields a system which will oscillate between two extreme states, either X or Y, which are dominated either by A or B. More complex networks can yield more complex state spaces.

Source: Donald E. Ingber, Sui Huang, A complex systems approach to understand how cells control their shape and make cell fate decisions. In *Encyclopedia of Genetics, Genomics, Proteomics and Bioinformatics*. Edited by Lynn Jorde, Peter Little, Mike Dunn and Shankar Subramaniam, Copyright © 2005 John Wiley & Sons, Ltd

balance. However, as we model this system over time, it reveals an apparently paradoxical result. In contrast to our expectations, in the top right panel we see that, far from an equivalence between the two states, the system ultimately converges on either one or another extreme stable configuration (minimum energy states) state X and state Y. State X is characterized by low A/ high B concentrations, while state Y has the opposite configuration. Despite the apparent balance in feedback mechanisms mediating each circuit, one component, either A or B, must ultimately dominate over time. Why do the components not balance each other, and what makes one gain an "advantage" over the other?

This rather confounding result seems to fly in the face of a structuralist perspective on biological determinism. Here we have a system with a perfectly designed structure for balance, and yet its ultimate functional fate is inevitably *imbalanced*—it ends in either A or B having a much higher concentration. This discrepancy emerges from the integration of the two principles we introduced previously: (1) the inevitable intervention of environmental dynamics and (2) the influence these will have over *time* on the dynamics of the system.

The role of the environment becomes inevitable because no system exists in isolation; whether this hypothetical biological circuit operates at the level of molecules, cells, circuits, organs, or the whole organism, it must ultimately involve some environmental input. This could involve the direct assimilation of environmental nutrients or toxicants; or, the perturbation might be driven by some change on another physiological level. And, this input might take the form of a deterministic process, for example some linear increase in the magnitude of nutrients or toxicants; or, it might be some stochastic (random) event, or a chaotic process.

But in whatever manner the environment should come to intrude upon this system, if at any given instant some perturbation should allow A to exceed B, even by a small amount, it will allow A to inhibit the activation of B, and thereby increase its own production through the positive feedback mechanism. Even an initially miniscule perturbation giving one circuit an advantage over the other will allow for a growing difference between them over time, until ultimately only one circuit dominates.[2] This process is very much akin to the seesaw found on any children's playground, but merely played out on the molecular level. This system appears balanced when both equally weighted parties are sitting on the ends of the apparatus, applying equal force; but, when one party applies a greater force than the other can reciprocate, the seesaw is doomed to end up tilted to one side.

Critically, the dynamics underlying the dependency between these systems, A and B, are impossible to generalize from the structural properties of either circuit, or from a measurement of either system at any given time. While the static topology of the system tells us something about what could in principle happen, the actual system dynamics can only become apparent by studying the systems over time. And, importantly, these not only will depend on the interdependencies between the elements of the system, A and B, but are also interdependent to the nature of environmental inputs to this system.

The bottom panel of Figure 4.1 generalizes this concept to a larger network with many more elements; rather than two interdependent circuits, we now model the interactions of a larger number of agents. One might suppose the increased complexity of this system would yield a corresponding increase in the diversity of conceivable outcomes; but, again counterintuitively, the bottom right panel of Figure 4.1 reveals an incredibly low number of possible stable states, corresponding to three possible outcomes in the valleys of the potential energy field. This drastic limitation of the possible configurations due to mutual correlation is both a general statistical law and great news for any scientist because we do not need to know the entirety of the underlying connectivity structure to predict the system's behavior; rather, we only need to measure the underlying dynamics on a sample of the state space.

The theoretical discussion so far tells us that considering *time* when looking at connections between systems may allow us to resolve some of the problems that are plaguing environmental sciences, specifically this increasing ocean of correlation with no sight of reconciling the complexity into a clear answer that tells us which state (health or disease) the system is heading toward.

Sensitive Dependence on Initial Conditions and the "n-Body Problem"

In the example discussed thus far we sought to emphasize several points. First, an examination of interdependency between two systems must involve an exploration of the processes and dynamics that connect these systems (i.e., the biodynamic interface). These emerge through a *temporal* exploration of system dynamics rather than an examination of static associations. Second, we sought to emphasize that interdependencies between any two systems inherently unfold across a broader network of relationships, both between an organism and its environment and between different levels of organization within the organism.

The latter focus is a major barrier in relating any given system to another; we are immediately challenged in defining what exactly we mean by "a system." We could define any one person as a biological system, for example, but this system inevitably includes a multitude of subsystems; for example, the cardiac system, central and peripheral nervous systems, pulmonary systems, and so on. And are not these systems, themselves, assembled from a variety of smaller systems—organs, circuits, valves, and chambers, which are themselves aggregates of muscle fibers, neurons, and specialized cells; and further, proteins, macromolecules, and ions? We thus find in every system that there are multiple levels of organization, from the simple to the unimaginably complex, and at every level of organization we find a different set of rules governing interactions within and between different levels (a thread we will pick up again in Chapter 6). To understand how these processes relate to the environment, we must understand how environmental inputs—themselves spanning macro- and micro-scale levels—are integrated and transmitted from one level to another.

Box 4.1 Biodynamic Field Hypothesis

The biodynamic interface conjecture—the idea at the core of Environmental Biodynamics—defines the nature of the connections between complex systems. Related to that is the question: *Why are we connected?* The biodynamic field hypothesis represents the beginnings of a journey to answer that question.

To convey this hypothesis let me (Arora) start with the story of an eye-opening conversation that I had with one of the other authors of this book, Alessandro Giuliani. I visited Alessandro in Rome and he took me for a walk that lasted about two hours; we visited places not popular on the tourist map, including the beautiful hidden medieval cloister of Santi Quattro Coronati. Alessandro has a knack for conveying the enormity of the history behind parts of Rome that many visitors would pass by without a second glance. Sitting down for lunch in a café that could barely hold 10 people, I asked Alessandro how the environment and human physiology are connected. He put forth an analogy that resonated with me. Being the kind of person who often makes a point by asking a question, Alessandro asked me how it was possible for his cellphone to connect to mine. There is a tendency to imagine some "thing," we often call it a "signal," leaving Alessandro's phone and reaching mine, very much like the toxic metal lead leaving the environment, being ingested or inhaled, entering our bloodstream, and then reaching our brains to induce an IQ deficit. But this is not entirely correct. The main reason one cellphone can connect with another is because both cellphones exist in a *field*. Without this electromagnetic field that connects the phone to towers and satellites, nothing from one cellphone can reach any other phone. It would be like screaming in the vacuum of deep space: No one is going to hear you. Instead, consider that all cellphones are embedded in a mesh and are already connected, but when one cellphone user needs to call another, the specific thread that links the two phones is activated.

In the same manner as cellphones in our analogy, humans are embedded in a field that includes our environment and other humans. This field is not flat but in fact is multidimensional. Imagine yourself immersed in a gel, where every part of the gel is connected to every other part. Extending this logic, it is also correct to say that you are connected to every other part, sometimes directly, sometimes through intervening components. This gel is not static; rather, it is constantly moving, and this movement has rhythmic components as well as chaotic dynamics in parts—that is to say, this field we are immersed in is itself *biodynamic*.

At the time of writing this book, this line of thought remains very much a hypothesis that needs further work to confirm its validity. It is our hope that by sharing this idea here, other scientists will join us in developing this further.

In other fields of science, the dependence of a given system's operation on interactions between its constituent parts, and with interdependent systems, is an old and well-recognized issue. The earliest articulations of this challenge are referred to as the "three-body problem;" or, more recently, and in reference to more complex systems, the "n-body problem" (we had briefly alluded to this in Chapter 3). This problem emerges in predicting the actions of multiple interacting components involved in a complex system; for example, the simultaneous movement of the sun, the earth, and the moon. The challenge here is that, much like the integrated levels of a biological system, the trajectory of each "body" in the three-body system (here: earth, moon, sun) is dependent on the trajectory of every other body. If any one body could be made to somehow "hold still" (or, in a gravitational system, stop exerting its mass on the other bodies), we might be able to determine the actions of the others; but, inevitably, the interdependence of three complex systems makes this problem intractable to solve (or at least, very difficult to solve, in light of recent advances in statistical physics that have broken new ground in addressing these challenges).[3]

To give you an idea of the complexity introduced by adding another body to a simple system, let's look again at a regular single pendulum with one spherical body at the end of an arm, as we did in Figure 3.2 in Chapter 3. That is a two-body scenario (the fixed end of the pendulum being the other "body"), and so a double pendulum as we have previously shown (Figure 3.3 in Chapter 3) is a three-body scenario. Unlike two-body problems, there is no closed-form solution (for example, the circle in Figure 3.2, panel C, is a closed form). Rather, the solution is far more elusive and can vary vastly due to small changes in initial conditions.

At the end of the 19th century, the mathematician and physicist Henri Poincaré demonstrated the existence of rather strange-appearing trajectories for three-body systems. In doing so, he discovered the concept of "sensitive dependence on initial conditions." With certain precise initial conditions, the three-body problem yields various patterns of simple, sometimes symmetrical and other times asymmetrical behavior. The pictures in Figure 4.2 show some of the possible repetitive orbits of a three-body system consisting of an idealized planet moving in the plane of a pair of stars that are in a perfect elliptical orbit.[4] These are among the earliest demonstrations of deterministic chaos, which describes a system with extraordinary sensitivity to initial conditions that is nonetheless not random in its motion (even though we may not be able to predict where it is headed).

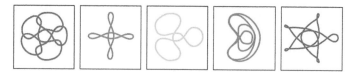

Figure 4.2 Orbits of the third body in a three-body system in which the other two bodies are in perfect elliptical orbit on a plane. Note that they are both regular and irregular; that is, discrete structures emerge, but these are highly sensitive (and therefore difficult to predict) to initial conditions.

Source: Wolfram, S. (2018). Notes for Chapter 7: Mechanisms in Programs and Nature, Section: Chaos Theory and Randomness from Initial Conditions. In *A New Kind of Science*, p. 972. © 2021 Stephen Wolfram, LLC. https://www.wolframscience.com.

Our examples might seem abstract and far from the topic of environmental medicine, but on the contrary they provide a well-delineated mathematical framework toward which environmental health has already begun to advance. The critical notion that emerged from Poincaré's work, and from later advancements by Edward Lorenz,[5] was the notion of a critical *dependence on initial conditions*, which predates and encompasses the developmental origins of health and disease (DoHAD) hypothesis that currently prevails in environmental epidemiology, which posits the origins of adult disease in early life dysregulation. As in the orbits of a strange attractor, the DoHAD perspective emphasizes how a small change in input in the early stages of a process can result in a large change in the system's ultimate trajectory—here, healthy development, rather than orbital trajectory. Through this lens, recent innovations in epidemiological practice, such as the focus on critical windows of vulnerability during development, are merely special cases of a sensitivity to initial conditions implicit to an n-body problem. Moreover, the relationship of our environment with our physiology is *never* a "two-body" problem but rather a complex manifold of nested n-body problems.

Let us take a step back and link what we have discussed here with other ideas introduced earlier in the book. As environmental health scientists, we are adept at asking *what* our environmental exposures are (for example, "what pesticides are in our food?"), *how intense* they are ("what is my blood lead level?"), and *how frequently* we experience those environmental exposures ("how often do you drink alcohol?"). Those lines of inquiry are standard structural approaches. However, we have thus far argued in this book that environmental health research would benefit from adding functional approaches to study our physiology, our environment, and their interdependence. Thus, we environmental health scientists must reflect on this point—when examining data on environmental exposures and their health impacts, we have to also ask questions such as the following:

1. What are the temporal dynamics—the periodic orbits, convergence, or bifurcation—of the systems involved with this environmental exposure and its assimilation into our physiology?

2. What is the complex pattern made by our biological systems (the "n-bodies")?

3. And how is that pattern perturbed by the addition of environmental factors (so now it's an "n + m body problem," where "m" denotes the environmental factors)?

Questions such as these need to be asked as often and answered with the same rigor as questions that pertain to the concentration and duration of exposure to any environmental factor. Furthermore, we suggest moving away from the notion of an equilibrium state where systems are constrained to stasis, or to a limited range of motion, because systems do not operate in isolation. Characterizing their dynamics requires a different mathematical framework than the statistical approaches currently employed. More profoundly, it requires a fundamental shift in the nature of the questions we ask about biological systems, and the interdependencies among them.

Incorporating Dynamic Interdependence in Environmental Medicine (Case Study)

Continuing with our studies on autism spectrum disorder, we have so far seen that by moving away from the structural approach to the more functional approaches (as discussed in Chapter 3), we were able to find a stable and reproducible signal that allowed us to distinguish children with and without autism spectrum disorder.[6,7] We now ask, in this chapter, how we can gain further insight into the biological mechanisms underlying this disorder by considering the system as a whole, and leveraging the multiple levels of organization in the interface mediating the individual and their environment. One approach we have developed to achieve this is based on the established methods of network analysis, which will be immediately familiar to anyone who has had digital social networking inflicted upon them.

To understand how this works, consider, as an analogy, any given individual in a digital social network, and the connections or "friends" they form within that network. Some individuals will form hundreds or thousands of connections, while others form very few; some individuals will find they have connections in common, while others are discrete. To understand these relationships, we might examine the network as a whole, in terms of characterizing the general pattern of connections, or we might focus on differences between individuals in terms of the number or types of connections they form. However, these dots and lines showing the connections are static; what if the connections and the entities being connected were dynamic? Like the sounds of musical instruments intermingling with each other, each time a new "friend" was added to your network, their musical contribution would be assimilated and the whole ensemble would evolve to sound different.

We applied a conceptually similar approach to characterize the biodynamic interfaces involved in elemental metabolism and their role in autism spectrum disorder. So far in this journey we had applied standard dynamical methods such as recurrence analysis (which is described in the appendix), with which we could characterize the complexity of periodic processes involved in various biodynamic interfaces; complexity in zinc and copper assimilation, for instance. But what about how they are interconnected? While those analyses effectively capture interdependencies between two metabolic pathways, they fail to place these in the context of the myriad other pathways that are simultaneously active and most likely interdependent as well. In a sense, where our prior analysis captured the orbital interdependencies between the earth and the moon, here we seek to characterize the wider solar system. You see, although we have looked at how zinc and copper orbits influence each other (just like one planet's orbit influences that of another), we haven't considered how all the various interfaces that regulate elemental assimilation are *interdependent* (that is, how the solar system moves as a whole).

An example of this approach is shown in Figure 4.3. Here, we want to give you a bird's-eye view of the network of biodynamic interfaces. This is a snapshot of a network that "hums" because each of its component parts are in constant motion. Here, each node of the network—each black dot where multiple lines meet—reflects a measure of dynamic complexity in a given elemental pathway (that is, the interface mediating the assimilation of that element in the body). You needn't read each of the labels on the graph, nor do you need to trace the path of each line; just know that stronger connections (higher correlations) are represented as thicker lines and weaker connections

Prenatal Recurrence networks in NT children

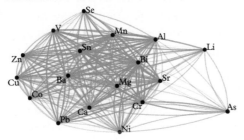

Prenatal Recurrence networks in ASD children

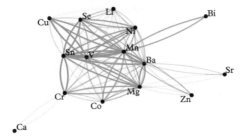

Figure 4.3 Dynamic connections in the metabolic trajectories of essential elements and toxic metals. The top graph shows the network of elemental dynamics in neurotypical (NT) children. In children with autism spectrum disorder (ASD; bottom graph), the network is fragmented, with fewer and generally weaker connections. Graph nodes are labeled with the chemical symbol of the element measured; in this case, we characterize periodic entropy in each pathway over time. Lines and corresponding line thicknesses reflect the strength of correlations between each pathway.

as thinner lines. At a glance it is immediately evident that, in children with autism spectrum disorder (bottom panel), interdependent dynamics are relatively sparse compared to that observed in healthy children (top panel). This physical nature of the problem here is the same as the one we described in the "molecular seesaw" examples in Figure 4.1—a change in wiring architecture, even a small one, will lead down a path to a "phenotypic state" (such as the valleys in Figure 4.1) that is very different from the state that would exist if there were no change in the wiring architecture.

So far, we have studied interdependence across one level, that of molecular networks. Does dynamic interconnectedness exist at the level of an organ's functioning? Furthermore, do biodynamic interfaces connect processes at different levels of organization, for example from molecular processes to whole organs to the level of an individual? To answer this, we analyzed the brain functioning of children enrolled in the autism twin study in Sweden using functional magnetic resonance neuroimaging (or fMRI as it is commonly known). fMRI measures brain activity by detecting changes associated with blood flow (and once again our collaborators led by Dr. Sven Bölte collected these data); regions of the brain that are more strongly activated will recruit a corresponding increase in blood flow.

fMRI signals are typically analyzed through the lens of correlation matrices that profile connectivity between different regions in various states, or through subsequent analyses applied to these correlations. In contrast, in our approach we sought to characterize activity in the brain in the same manner as we had studied the assimilation of environmental elemental exposures; that is, through the reconstruction of an underlying attractor system, and through the analysis of functional dynamics in the attractor (recall that we have discussed attractors in Chapter 3). The results of this analysis are shown in Figure 4.4. Without going into too much technical detail, what you are seeing in the panel on the left is the topography of the brain's function (not its structure) over time in the form of a potential energy landscape. This reflects the stability and complexity of a given attractor system, and the likelihood that a system will remain in a persistent orbit. As with attractors describing elemental metabolism, the valleys here represent periods of stability and the peaks are tipping points where brain function moves from one state to another (note also the similarity in the "valleys" in these real-life data with the hypothetical example

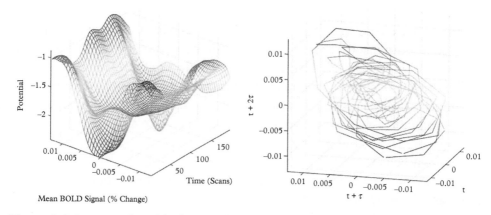

Figure 4.4 Attractor dynamics in neural networks. Left panel shows the potential energy landscape derived from an analysis of default mode network BOLD signals. At right, the Takens reconstruction of the attractor system.

in Figure 4.1 showing the valleys where the circuit is destined to move toward). In the right panel, we show the typical Takens reconstruction of the attractor system, as discussed in Chapter 3; note the circular orbit, emphasizing both the periodic dynamics dominating this system and an underlying drift in the dynamic over time.

We had thus characterized the dynamics of the physiological system of interest (neural connectivity), but do dynamic interfaces connect systems operating at different levels? To answer this, we analyzed the dynamics of elemental assimilation (specifically, zinc and copper dynamics) with the dynamics we had just observed in brain functioning as measured by fMRI. Just as we found that dysregulation of the zinc–copper biodynamic interface was linked to diagnosis of autism spectrum disorder, we found that zinc–copper dynamics were also predictive of dynamics in brain functioning, which itself was linked to autism-related traits. What this showed was that dynamic interfaces connect systems not only at one level (molecule to molecule, for example) but *across* levels (molecular orbits to organ functioning to organism-level behavior). The properties of dynamic interfaces thus appear to propagate across multiple levels of organization, which presents a new avenue for studies exploring the interaction of our environment with our health.

The advantage of applications like these is that they leverage both the fine-scale dynamics characterized in the biodynamic interface and the organization of interdependent systems, which may yield emergent properties not apparent in the analysis of a single given system. More broadly, these approaches seek to provide holistic measures of how the body and the environment are functioning in unison at multiple levels of biological organization, each interdependent on another, and they include *time* as a central feature of this interdependence. This also has broader consequences because, if we take interdependence seriously, we are forced to drastically rethink our attitude toward current approaches to causality and explanation in biology. The prophetic intuition of Warren Weaver of the existence of "three kingdoms of science" that we introduced in Chapter 1 are now even more evident—in the realm of organized complexity, any useful explanation needs to focus on the *time-varying dynamics of connections*.

The vision and hope of Environmental Biodynamics is to integrate these approaches in our systemic assessment of human health, toward the goal of predicting, diagnosing, and characterizing human disease more swiftly, effectively, and accurately. Rather than providing a blood sample and waiting to find if essential elements and toxins are within or outside some idealized numerical range, we should be developing dynamic assessments that determine if our physiological systems and the environment within which they exist are properly synchronized, both at the level of discrete pathways that may be implicated in a given disease and at the level of holistic interdependencies that maintain and organize health. Environmental Biodynamics provides a roadmap to achieve this.

We offer the following example as practical demonstration of the clinical utility of this perspective. As we alluded to in Chapter 3, the ultimate goal of these advances is to yield tools that allow us to describe, explain, and predict the emergence of disease. And, the insights emphasized here, and previously in Chapter 3, propel us toward that goal. That is, we have described health not in a static context of concentrations or linear correlations, but rather by measuring physiological dynamics through the lens of *organization*, and connected these processes from the level of environmental assimilation (the intake and metabolism of a chemical exposure) to dynamics in neural connectivity. Further, we have explained differences in neurodevelopmental outcomes by identifying how these dynamics differ in neurotypical individuals, and those with neurodevelopmental disorders. What we have yet to offer in this story is the extension of this perspective to predictive framework.

To achieve this, we return to our initial study which focused on characterizing dynamics in the assimilation of essential elements during early life, including prenatal and early childhood development. As explained previously, we leveraged advances in laser ablation and mass spectrometry to reconstruct zinc and copper concentrations at high temporal resolution throughout development; but, rather than focus on the intensity of zinc and copper we used methods of attractor reconstruction and recurrence quantification analysis to measure determinism, entropy, and periodicity (rhythms) in the assimilation of these elements over time. As noted, this descriptive analysis enabled us to identify and explain differences between children with typical and atypical (ASD-related) neurodevelopment. As our next step, consistent with the goals of Environmental Biodynamics, we sought to leverage these measures to develop a *predictive* tool that would have clear clinical utility.

Recall that, although the retrospective environmental data analyzed in this study related to prenatal and early childhood time periods, the participating children were actually much older by the time of our analysis, and in fact had already undergone clinical screening throughout their childhood. As such, we had detailed records as to which children developed typically, and which children developed ASD. We thus sought to ask: can we use the dynamics measured at the level of biodynamic interface in early life to predict later health outcomes?

To achieve this, we constructed a machine learning model (in actuality, an ensemble of several models) which leveraged data derived from our analysis of zinc-copper attractors. We "trained" these models—in simple terms, "teaching" them about relationships between dynamics and case status—on one subset of our data; then, used the trained models to make predictions of case status on another subset of our data that we had never seen (that is, a blinded analysis). Our results indicated a profound insight: using only information about the nature and organization of interfaces in elemental metabolism, we were 90% accurate in predicting the emergence of ASD *years in advance of any behavioral symptoms*. In essence, this study provides an initial demonstration of the feasibility and utility of leveraging Environmental Biodynamics for ASD; but, more generally, this approach provides the roadmap needed to generalize Environmental Biodynamics to explain a broader spectrum of health and disease.

Chapter 4 Summary

That complex systems would interact directly seems so obvious a notion that we suspect most wouldn't even give it a thought (even though it is incorrect, as we have proposed). Throughout the history of science, this has often been the case for other seemingly mundane observations, such as an apple falling from a tree—"Well, of course, apples fall from trees; that's what apples do" is the sort of thinking that remains pervasive, even in science. And for whatever reason, the everyday common-ness of such events makes them seem to lack any underlying importance. But to the contrary, we have found something special in common, everyday, mundane and obvious observations. We have found that complex systems *cannot* interact directly, nor can they exist in isolation. Rather, interdependencies between one system and another are propagated through temporal dynamics that emerge through the integration of the system's properties and environmental changes.

In Chapters 2 and 3, we have discussed how moving from a structural to a functional worldview requires us to embrace the constantly changing nature of our physiology and our environment. But *constant change* does not mean that everything is random or that we are on unsteady ground; rather, we have shown that there is shape to this change and have called it "structured dynamism" (Chapter 3). This change is a key component of the biodynamic interfaces that facilitate the interaction between systems. We have taken another step and shown that our understanding of biodynamic interfaces is dependent on our temporal perspective. In other words, the picture we see depends on where *and when* we are (Chapter 2). In both Chapters 2 and 3, we have for the most part treated the biodynamic interfaces as independent entities. That is obviously not the case—biodynamic interfaces are connected to each other and, as always, we must remember to place *time* at the center of these connections. These connections are not like networks of roads that are static; they are more like an ensemble of musicians who are constantly in motion and their joint motion (their music) creates a whole that has meaning.

References

1. Ingber, D. E., & Huang, S. (2005). A complex systems approach to understand how cells control their shape and make cell fate decisions. In L. B. Jorde, P. F. R. Little, M. J. Dunn, & S. Subramaniam (Eds.), *Encyclopedia of Genetics, Genomics, Proteomics and Bioinformatics*. Wiley. https://doi.org/10.1002/047001153X.g308208

2. Huang, S. (2009). Reprograming cell fates: reconciling rarity with robustness. *Bioessays* 31, 546–560, doi:10.1002/bies.200800189.

3. Stone, N. C., & Leigh, N. W. C. (2019). A statistical solution to the chaotic, non-hierarchical three-body problem. *Nature* **576**, 406–410, https://doi.org/10.1038/s41586-019-1833-8.

4. Wolfram, S. (2018). A New Kind of Science. Wolfram Media.

5. Motter, A. E., & Campbell, D. K. (2013). Chaos at fifty. *Physics Today* **66**(5), 27–33.

6. Austin, C., et al. (2019). Dynamical properties of elemental metabolism distinguish attention deficit hyperactivity disorder from autism spectrum disorder. *Translational Psychiatry* **9**(1), 238, doi:10.1038/s41398-019-0567-6.

7. Curtin, P., et al. (2018). Dynamical features in fetal and postnatal zinc-copper metabolic cycles predict the emergence of autism spectrum disorder. *Science Advances* **4**(5), eaat1293, doi:10.1126/sciadv.aat1293.

5

The Geometry of Health

Patterns, Structures, Forms, and Constraints

Dimensions of Health and Disease

The most humbling challenge in studying human health is also perhaps the most easily overlooked: We don't really have a definitive indicator of overall "health." As a concept health is not so easily pinned down for the scientist as, say, the idea of the cell, which might be thought of as "all the stuff within the cell membrane" (at least, in an animal cell). Part of the problem in approaching health is that we lack any clear boundary around which we might say someone *is* or *is not* healthy; would we be referring to the person as a whole in defining their health, or specifically to their discrete parts? If the former, then an otherwise healthy person might suffer from an infected hangnail or a fractured arm, for example, as their other systems remain intact; if the latter, one would require that the whole person be absent of any sort of defect, and by that standard surely almost none of us are healthy. And, in both cases, we have arrived at our definition of health not by identifying something that is present—that is, some aspect of *healthiness*—but rather by *failing to detect* the presence of something else—*sickness*. If we can define and detect one, why not the other?

But, of course, there are other aspects to human health than the mere presence or absence of sickness, and perhaps in consideration of these factors the nature of human health may become clearer. Resilience, for example, has nothing to do with the presence or absence of current injury or disease, but rather describes a capacity to resist sickness or injury, and/or the robust recovery from some departure from health. As well, independent of the presence

Environmental Biodynamics. Manish Arora and Paul Curtin with Austen Curtin, Christine Austin, and Alessandro Giuliani, Oxford University Press. © Oxford University Press 2022. DOI: 10.1093/oso/9780197582947.003.0005

of or resistance to illness or disease, our conception of health includes some aspect of functionality to it. That is, two people, equally free of illness or injury, might be thought to differ in their healthiness on the basis of their fitness, physical and emotional endurance, and even personal attitudes.

Each of these perspectives on health is necessary to study the interaction between our environment and our health, but when considered in isolation each is inadequate. Every one of these measures provides just a single dimension along which health may vary, much as a measurement of height or width can only provide a single dimension describing the shape of an object. And, as in any complex system, in considering health we must determine what dimensions are needed to fully capture this concept and apply it to useful medical and scientific applications. Here, we outline how Environmental Biodynamics seeks to leverage a multitude of functional dimensions to describe human health in terms of dynamic patterns and forms.

Patterns, Structures, Forms, and Constraints in Biological Systems

Dimensionality is an inherently exciting concept to any fan of science fiction, implying some capacity to explore or transcend some heretofore-unknown aspects of reality. In the practical application of science, however, the operational meaning of "dimensions" is more prosaic, referring to the number of different coordinates you need to unequivocally define a point. We typically describe the topography of the world around of us along the dimensions of height, width, and depth—and we might be interested in how these features vary along a fourth dimension, *time*. Any of these measures, or indeed any single variable along which a system may vary, can be considered a discrete, singular dimension. The challenge posed to the scientist, of course, is to identify what dimensions are necessary to describe, explain, predict, and/or control a given system. This might include anything from the familiar spatial dimensions to measures of functional performance, such as heart rate, blood pressure, or response to social stress, for example, or any of the countless ways the body and its operations might be measured. In clinical medicine, the challenge becomes the identification of dimensions that allow us to characterize a system's function sufficiently to make accurate predictions of its future state (is it heading toward disease?) or to alter its trajectory to a desirable state (return it to health).

This problem is generally challenging in the broad context of biology but is especially so in the specific application of human health and its relationship to the environment, because the question we are asking is: *What dimensions, exactly, are needed to characterize and define the interface mediating a biological system's interaction with the environment?* The spatial dimensions of height, width, and length may be useful in describing the location and shape of a system but are surely inadequate in describing its structure: They ignore its mass, for instance, and related properties such as its density, as well as a whole host of physical attributes (color, elemental composition, conductivity, for example). Worse, these few dimensions are entirely inadequate in characterizing *function*—two systems of similar composition may have vastly different functional capacities. Remember, for example, the oft-quoted finding that humans and chimpanzees share the vast majority of our genome and, as well, from a structural genetic perspective, that both of these great apes have quite a lot in common with a bumblebee, a slime mold, and a banana.

In a *functional* reality, the organization of life is very different. From the simplest of biological entities, at the levels of cells and organelles, to the organization of complex organisms, biological systems cascade across a messy, multidimensional manifold from which functionality emerges—a process not easily derived from a summary measure of any singular dimensional feature. Furthermore, which dimensions are relevant to the biological process at hand are a function of the level of biological organization—molecular, cellular, systemic, organismal—and the context under which the analysis is being undertaken. Minor temperature fluctuations may be a critical determinant of chemical and molecular interactions in the cell, for example, but might not be relevant to predict the behavior of a whole organism.

What measures can possibly summarize a biological system, then, if any given dimension is by itself inadequate, and any given multitude of biological dimensions that are likely to be relevant will inevitably vary according to the system and research question? We propose that the answer to this question lies in understanding the underlying patterns and forms from which the data arise. Consider, as an example, the oval shadow depicted in Figure 5.1 (left panel). This is the representation of what scientists everywhere ponder over persistently—data that originate from a scientific exercise in observing a natural phenomenon (for example, levels of nutrients and toxicants in people's blood, resting heart rate, gene expression, or any other biological measurement). In other words, this is some biological dimension that we have measured or observed. Let us ask a seemingly simple question: How can we use the

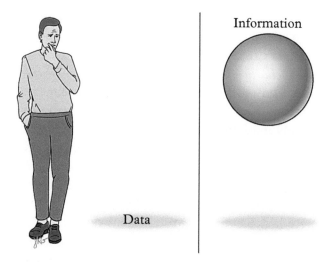

Figure 5.1 Data collected on human health or our environment are representations of multidimensional processes. In our analogy, if the ellipsoid shadow is the data that we gather during a scientific exercise, then we can infer that the higher-dimensional processes generating the information behind the data are constrained to a corresponding shape—a sphere in our example. In this manner the analysis of underlying forms permits a deeper understanding of complex biological processes that are behind our scientific observations.

structure of these data to understand the process that generated this pattern? The organization of the observed data—the circular shape of the shadow— suggests that the origins of this two-dimensional piece of information (this shadow) must reflect some property of its three-dimensional source (right panel). We can infer from the generally ellipsoid shape of the shadow, for example, that the source of the data was most likely also ellipsoid; were the shadow cast from another source, like a tree or a person, its form would be constrained to resemble those patterns.

The derivation of an underlying form from the pattern we observe leads us to deeper questions on the nature of forms, such as: Are there underlying rules driving the forms that impact function in biological and environmental systems (in the same way that the shadow cast by a sphere will be constrained to an ellipsoid shape)? To begin to answer this question, let us consider one of the simplest geometrical forms, the triangle. Figure 5.2 depicts three triangles of different sizes; these triangles are considered "similar" in that the angles in all three triangles are identical. The lengths of the edges of the triangles

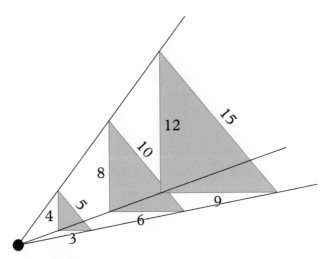

Figure 5.2 All the triangles are a different size, but the length of their sides can be characterized by studying the constraints applied by the similar angles. Furthermore, the shape of unobserved triangles can also be estimated by understanding the nature of the constraints.

nonetheless differ, but despite this there is a constancy in the pattern of their organization because they keep their mutual ratios, relating the lengths of each side, strictly invariant. The constraints in the underlying form of each triangle—specifically, the invariance in the angles—thus imposes a constraint on each of the three edges that prevents them from varying independently. Each change in one edge goes with a particular change in the other two. These constraints allow the generation of an infinite array of triangles of varying sizes, but the constraints in their underlying forms will impose a common pattern to the size ratios of each triangle's sides. This then leads to obvious questions that are relevant to understanding health and disease: *Are there such constraints operating in biological systems? Can the exploration of underlying constraints inform our understanding of biological dimensionality? And does the violation of such constraints lead to ill health?*

Because these questions are so fundamental, a major focus of computational biology has been to identify the underlying forms that are present in biological systems and to use these to characterize and predict the patterns we observe in the biological world—to understand, as in our first example, what is the true source of the shapes we see in our data. A study conducted 60 years ago by Jolicoeur and Mosimann provides a clear illustration of this process in a seemingly unlikely source—the strikingly colorful patterns of the painted turtle's shell.[1] Seeking to understand the nature of diversity in this species, which, ultimately, will determine how that species adapts and responds to selective challenges, the authors of that study collected samples from the ponds and lakes in North America and Europe to measure both the size and shape of *Chrysemis picta* (the painted turtle) shells. Figure 5.3 shows a typical carapace of the painted turtle seen from above. As in the hypothetical shadow or the calculated triangle, the carapace of the turtle can be easily characterized in spatial dimensions, in that it can be defined in terms of its length, width. and

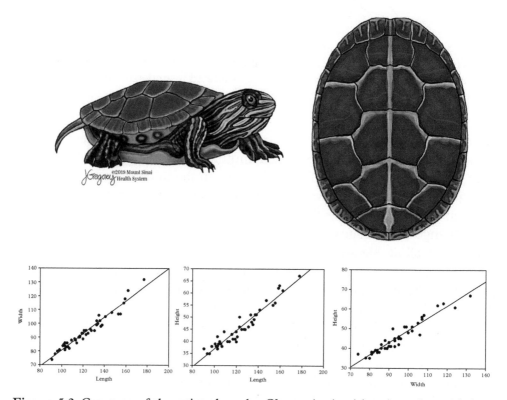

Figure 5.3 Carapace of the painted turtle, *Chrysemis pica* (above), and correlations among dimensional measures (height, width, and length) of the turtle's shell (below). Each of these dimensions is strongly related to the other, just as the triangle's sides were (the correlation coefficients exceeded 0.95 in each comparison).

Source: Jolicoeur P, Moisimann JE (1960). Size and shape variation in the painted turtle. A principal component analysis. Growth. 24. PMID: 13790416. https://citeseerx.ist.psu.edu/viewdoc/download?doi=10.1.1.454.279&rep=rep1&type=pdf.

height. But are the dimensions of a turtle's shell constrained by an underlying *form* as the ratios of the triangles' sides were in our earlier example?

To test this, the authors of that study used a simple associative statistical method, correlational analysis, to evaluate the constraints that the three dimensions of the turtle's shell impose on each other. In Figure 5.3 (bottom panel) we show data from the original study that verifies the importance of mutual dependency in dimensions. In the plots, each point corresponds to a specific turtle, and each axis is one of the three dimensions measured on an individual animal. These results indicate that each dimension of the turtle's shell is highly correlated with another dimension; a shell that is long will also be wide, and a shell that is thick ("height") will also be long. From an evolutionary and ecological perspective, of course, this makes sense that length, width, and height must co-vary and constrain each other in order for the shell as a whole to remain functional and serve its adaptive purpose.

But from another perspective, focusing on the relationship between pattern and form, this example illustrates that biological systems must follow the same simple logic by which we describe, explain, and predict the world in mathematical terms, seeking always to understand the structure that organized the form of our data. In fact, this simple approach can be extended further through a variety of mathematical techniques, such as principal component analysis (PCA; see Box 5.1 for description). These approaches, called *dimensionality-reduction* techniques, seek to explicitly achieve the goal of identifying underlying forms and constraints by reconstructing a new dimensional space derived from the initial measures of the system. In essence, given the observed correlations among the three dimensions of data, this approach seeks to reconstruct the other two dimensions starting from only one due to the existence of a typical form that sets limits on how the three dimensions of the object can vary. For a simple biological pattern such as the growth of the turtle's shell, this might be accomplished by reconstructing a single underlying dimension; just as the ratio of sides reflects the constraints in the structure of similar triangles, this underlying dimension is representative of the typical pattern of growth in this species. Thus, in the same way that we use the size ratios of similar triangles to predict the shape of another similar triangle, the dimensions derived from techniques such as PCA can allow us to identify the underlying patterns that are predicted by the dimensions we observe in biological systems.

Our emphasis on forms and patterns, both in the abstract in relation to geometrical forms and in the practical example of the turtle's carapace, is to

---

Box 5.1 A Note on Principal Component Analysis

By far the most widespread method to reduce the number of measured dimensions to reveal which smaller subset carries enough information to predict the other ones is principal component analysis, a statistical technique developed by Karl Pearson in 1901, which seeks to identify underlying patterns that organize the variability in a given system.[2]

In essence, PCA is a mathematical procedure that transforms a number of correlated variables into a smaller number of uncorrelated variables called principal components (PCs). Each PC is composed of the weighted integration of the original variables, with each variable weighed more or less heavily on a given component. The first PC accounts for as much of the variability in the data as possible, and each succeeding component accounts for as much of the remaining variability. In practice, once we have identified the source for most of the variability, say 90%, we just focus on those characteristics (or dimensions) of the system.

In the case of the painted turtle, PCA identifies an underlying dimension; we call this dimension PC1, and it is the maximal length of the carapace. In this dataset this one measure, PC1, explained 98% of the total information present on the turtle's shell, and allowed for a one-dimensional estimation of the turtle's size by a global score encompassing the three dimensions (for those familiar with PCA, PC1 = 33.8*Length + 33.7*Width + 33.6*Height).

---

emphasize that biological measurements can be considered both (1) from the perspective of the actual measurements along a given dimension and (2) as tools to explore and define the underlying biological form. In our own research, we look for the existence of specific patterns in our data by looking for the presence of correlation structures—relationships between one measurement and another—in the hope that these reveal the shape of the health of a system or organ, and we will provide an example of this from our work on autism spectrum disorder (ASD) later in the chapter.

Discrete and Integrated Assessments of Biological Dimensionality

The challenge of identifying the relevant dimensions across which biological systems vary has consumed much of biological inquiry for the past century. More recently, the rise of -omics technologies, which allow characterization of biological systems from the levels of nucleotide sequences, epigenomic modifications, protein expression, and metabolomic processing, has accelerated this process tremendously in characterizing literally millions of dimensions across which biological systems adapt (and we remind the reader that the term "dimensions" as used here refers to characteristics or variables). The dream in these pursuits is to assemble a high-dimensional depiction of the biological system that describes, explains, and predicts the trajectory of a life form: its development, its mature phenotype, and its fate. In these analyses, each measure from an -omics analysis is being treated as a dimension. The reader at this point should be aware that these multiple dimensions are not independent of each other, and since we are speaking about "organisms" we are actually dealing with intermingled networks of correlations in both space and time allowing the system to work as an integrated whole (the "organized complexity" realm of Warren Weaver, as discussed in Chapter 1). We are actually dealing with *forms*, but, sadly enough, in much of scientific practice this very basic fact is almost entirely overlooked.

Achieving these high-dimensional descriptions has essentially proceeded along two different paths. In one approach, particularly common to genomics, metabolomics, and related fields, associative studies are used; genome-wide association studies (GWAS) in that context, but epigenomic-wide association study (EWAS) and metabolome-wide association study (MWAS) strategies have evolved in other -omics fields as well.[3-5] The premise of this approach is in considering each of the many thousands of -omic variables measured, which might reflect individual gene expression, epigenetic modification (e.g., DNA methylation), or metabolite concentration, and evaluating individual associations between these and some health-related or biological variable. The research question becomes, essentially, whether a given gene (or other -omic feature) relates to a given health outcome, and this question is then reiterated hundreds or thousands of times to profile the full system. Here, the concept of form is totally discarded—each single variable is a standalone bit of information we explore for its value in predicting some feature of interest (discriminating those with or without a disease, for example). There are of course many dozens, even hundreds, of variations along this theme, from the use of variable-selection methods to the integration of bioinformatics and related machine-learning and computational methods. But in general, here, we designate these as *discrete* approaches; that is, they seek to identify the role of a given dimension—say, the expression level of a gene—as considered in isolation.

Box 5.2 Constraints on Form Without Constraints on Diversity

Any keen observer of our world would have noticed that, of the infinite options available, nature tends to repeat certain forms, often at vastly different scales. Why is it that trees, the fine-scale branching structure of our lungs (from the bronchi to the bronchioles), and lightning strikes all share the same fundamental form, even though we would consider their origins to be entirely different? One reason for this is that such patterns optimize the function of a system while demanding less energy input during the formation and subsequent operations of the system. In other words, these patterns are highly efficient; in the case of lungs, the particular branching structure maximizes the transfer of oxygen from the lungs to the blood while using less energy than other organizational structures would require. At a deeper level of analysis, the answer to the question of why the universe repeats such patterns is that there are fundamental rules that underlie the organization of systems. Of particular relevance to our examples just mentioned are the rules that drive the formation of *fractals*. A simplified description of fractals is that they are geometric shapes whose parts resemble the whole. As such, when we zoom in to examine any component of a fractal, it resembles the bigger structure it is part of. Fractals are not the only rules that govern the form of systems in our universe but we mention them here specifically because they are among the more well-studied ones and, more importantly, they shed light on a seemingly counterintuitive assumption about "constraints"—that they restrict diversity. That is not true. Just like no two trees are identical but they all share a similar form, and this can also be said of snowflakes, lightning strikes, and countless entities in our universe, the presence of underlying rules and the constraints they apply does not limit the multitude of possible forms; rather, it asks them to share common features that make them efficient. This realization is very important to our work because, after all, we are proposing that complex systems can only interact via an operationally independent interface that applies constraints on what information is transferred between the interacting systems. Furthermore, as we will show later in this chapter, by characterizing the underlying forms we can provide a measure of health (or disease) that no singular measure of a dimension ever could.

A second general strategy for making sense of the breadth and diversity of biological dimensions relates back to the concepts of dimensionality reduction introduced earlier in this chapter. This approach begins with the same challenge as described in the association-wide study—that is, a vast array of biological dimensions, and a desire to understand them. But rather than analyze each dimension in isolation, here we seek to understand the structure of constraints and mutual correlations that relate each variable to another, and ultimately test how these constraints relate to health. In essence, returning to our initial example of the triangles' geometry, where the -omic-wide association study would test if the length of any given triangle side relates to an outcome, in this approach we test the significance of the ratio that links each side to the other two.

A diverse array of algorithms has been developed to achieve this, including the previously introduced PCA, but most follow the basic logic of seeking a smaller subset of dimensions that captures the variability observed across a larger set of dimensions. Some of the earliest and best-known examples of these approaches emerged in the psychological literature, particularly studies of personality and individual variability. The "Big 5" personality traits, in fact, offer a striking example of this approach.[6] These comprise the traits of openness, conscientiousness, extraversion, agreeableness, and neuroticism, each reflecting an underlying dimension across which a given individual's personality may vary. An individual's affinity for these traits is assessed through the administration of a personality survey, which poses many discrete questions to which the individual responds. Each of these may be considered a unique dimension on which a person is measured, and, from these dimensions of individual survey items, the five underlying primary dimensions of personality are derived. This is no different from the example of the turtle's shell. Here, too, we are trying to uncover the underlying form and the constraints applied to it because of its mutual covariance with other characteristics of the organism, just as the length of the turtle's shell varies with its width. The ultimate goal in such an approach, whether applied in big-data biological assays such as the genome or in psychological studies, is to identify an underlying pattern or structure in complex high-dimensional data.

In reality, these seemingly opposing perspectives, which seek to analyze biological relationships as either discrete entities or pattern-driven systems, are often integrated in practice or applied in parallel. Studies using dimensionality-reduction techniques might follow their analysis of principal components (derived dimensions) with an associative analysis to relate these underlying dimensions to health; or, likewise, studies using an association-wide approach to genomic data might be linking the discrete effect of various genes to some psychological construct derived through a dimensionality-reduction technique. These sorts of divisions can become particularly blurry in the context of exposure biology, where frequently we investigate the combined effect of multiple simultaneous exposures—an application referred to as mixtures modeling—where it is entirely plausible that the combined effect of multiple environmental exposures is greater than the individual effect of

Box 5.3 Structural and Functional Perspectives on Mechanism

Due to the many advances in -omic technologies that have allowed us to study human physiology at ever-finer spatial scales, the focus on "mechanism" has often taken a reductionist approach, tunneling deeper to discover molecular markers in the expectation that molecules would explain complex phenomena at all levels of observation, including at societal levels. As a consequence, in studies examining the interaction of the environment and human physiology, the search for mechanisms has taken the form of identifying molecules that may be up- or down-regulated along a pathway diagram. We provide an analogy here to convey why this approach has had limited success in providing consequential understanding of human–environment interactions.

In the figure below we show two systems interacting—System A is a human hand that will be transferring information to System B, a piece of paper. Under a reductionist approach, System A would be examined in ever-smaller spatial scales, from organ to tissue to cellular to the genetic level and, similarly, System B would be examined down to the molecular and ionic levels. However, neither analysis can predict the style of handwriting; nor, more profoundly, could either approach even begin to elucidate the language, or the meaning of what is written to a reader. To have an accurate measure of this transfer of information, it is necessary to examine the process-based (and, therefore, dynamic) interface that connects the two systems, which in this case is the process of writing. This does not mean that all that is ever written on the piece of paper is necessary. Rather, a small piece of handwriting can be used to deduce the style or pattern of handwriting produced by a person with remarkable detail, as is the case in forensic analysis. This seemingly mundane detail is important because during any scientific experiment examining system-to-system interactions, the whole set of information is never available; rather, the wider set is deduced from a small finite collection of data (i.e., the experimental data).

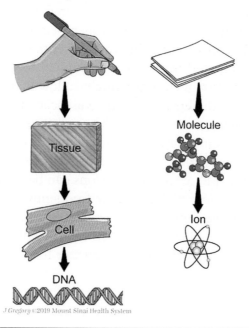

J Gregory ©2019 Mount Sinai Health System

any one exposure. Methodologies useful in these approaches can simultaneously leverage both associative and dimensionality-reduction techniques.

With Environmental Biodynamics we seek to engender a shift in how we approach and consider the "problem" of biological dimensionality. Beyond the fast-changing landscape of varying methodologies and approaches, the fundamental nature of how we approach and consider biological dimensionality needs to be reconsidered. While traditionally environmental health studies have embraced an associative or pattern-based analytical framework, we now must move to include measures and interpretations of "biological reality." This is the same scenario we alluded to earlier in Chapter 1—the difference between knowing *when* apple trees will shed their fruit versus understanding *why* an apple falls to the earth. One is *prediction*; the other is an *explanation*. In expanding the focus of environmental health science to a functional analysis of health, we also seek to return to a biologically driven analysis of the forms, constraints, and patterns that drive biological systems and ultimately human health. In the following example, we illustrate how the measurement of patterns extracted from elemental metabolism allowed us to identify underlying forms relating to the emergence of neurodevelopmental disorders.

Leveraging Patterns, Structures, Forms, and Constraints in Health Research (Case Study)

It would be reasonable to ask: *What is the practical use of a focus on underlying forms? How does it help a patient?* The answer is that it allows a powerful insight into human health that simply was not possibly from the perspective of discrete analyses of physiological parameters. We first demonstrated this when we were able to build an algorithm that allowed us to detect ASD with over 90% accuracy based on measurements of prenatal elemental dynamics (see Chapter 4).[7] We likewise showed how the dynamics underlying the assimilation of essential and toxic metals existed as temporal interdependent "networks," and in children with ASD, this interdependency was fragmented. Now, we extend this work by using the ideas presented in this chapter and ask the question: *What are the underlying "forms" in our data?* In the same way that the turtle's shell could be understood by measuring the relationship between the various dimensions of its form, and also the same manner in which people's questionnaire responses could be used to calculate the underlying forms of their personality, we wanted to know the underlying neurodevelopmental forms in the participants we were studying. It was one thing to distinguish children who had ASD from those who did not, but that is not the only type of neurodevelopmental disorder that exists.

The clearest example of this came in a recent follow-up analysis[7] of our ASD study in Sweden where we used this approach to distinguish not only those who have ASD from controls but also those who have attention-deficit/hyperactivity disorder (ADHD) and those who have both ASD and ADHD (i.e., those who are comorbid). In Figure 5.4, we show a method that shares some properties with PCA; it is called linear discrimination analysis and used not just one chemical measurement (such as the complexity of the zinc orbit, as discussed in Chapter 3) but rather over 300 properties of the essential and toxic metals we had measured and how the assimilation of these elements was interdependent (as discussed in Chapter 4). By doing so, we developed a multidimensional algorithm that distinguishes the underlying neurodevelopmental form of our participants, in the same manner as others have identified "personality types." Admittedly, much more work is to be done before we can apply this technology as a diagnostic tool for ASD or any other neurodevelopmental condition, but our purpose in highlighting it here is to show the promise of Environmental Biodynamics. Our vision is to integrate these approaches in our systemic assessment of human health, toward the goal of predicting, diagnosing, and characterizing human disease more swiftly, effectively, and accurately. Rather than providing a blood sample and waiting to find if levels of essential elements and toxins are within or outside some idealized numerical range, we should be developing dynamic assessments that determine if our physiological systems and the environment within which they exist are properly synchronized, both at the level of discrete pathways that may be implicated in a given disease and at the level of holistic interdependencies that maintain and organize health. Environmental Biodynamics provides a roadmap to achieve this.

Chapter 5 Summary

Our physiology and our environment do not "connect" with each other as would two electronic devices via a cable. Neither does the environment "pour" all its influence into us like a beaker transferring water into a cup. Rather, we

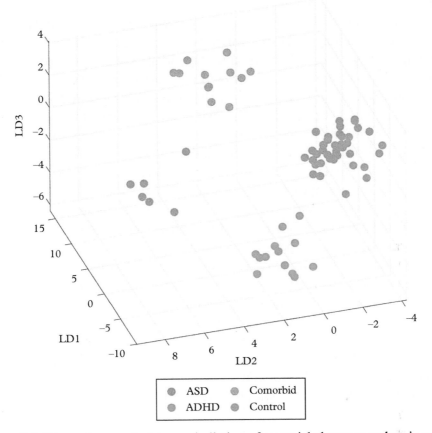

Figure 5.4 Dimensions underlying assimilation of essential elements and toxic metals in ASD. By studying the forms, patterns, and constraints of the dynamic nature of elemental assimilation, we were able to distinguish neurotypical children from those who had ASD, those who had ADHD, and those who had both these neurodevelopmental disorders.

have argued that these two complex systems cannot interact *directly*—that is the guiding idea at the center of Environmental Biodynamics. So, how then do we interact with our environment? We conjecture that our physiology and our environment both contribute to the formation of an interface, and by doing so they give rise to an intermediary that guides our interaction by letting some influences pass between the systems while restricting others. This intermediary is a process-based biodynamic interface.

In Chapter 3, we discussed how this interface is undergoing constant change, and to understand it, a first important step was to characterize the topography of this ever-changing interface, which we refer to as the "shape of change." In Chapter 4, we focused on the interdependence of systems on other systems, and how the connections between them are themselves dynamic. Here in Chapter 5, we further examine the dynamic nature of interfaces and start examining their characteristics. We posit that just as we might derive a multitude of dimensions to describe biological structure, so too are there many dimensions that describe the functional dynamics in how biological systems vary over *time*. Current environmental epidemiological methods used in analyzing data on our environment and our physiology treat each measure as if it were an independent dimension, much like a carpenter measuring the height, width, or length of a piece of furniture. However, because there are processes underlying our physiological development, we have constraints applied to the forms that we and our environment can take, just as in the case of the carapace of the turtle. Knowledge of these can be harnessed to identify the primary dimensions along which we must characterize the systems under study. By doing this we were able to take an important first step in operationalizing Environmental Biodynamics for clinical application. We showed how our work on ASD went from being a correlative study to one that has the potential to detect health disorders many years before any clinical signs appear. We're not there yet, but the tools are now available to achieve that.

References

1. Jolicoeur, P., & Mosimann, J. E. (1960). Size and shape variation in the painted turtle: a principal component analysis. *Growth* **24**, 339–354, https://citeseerx.ist.psu.edu/viewdoc/download?doi=10.1.1.454.279&rep=rep1&type=pdf.
2. Pearson, K. (1901). On lines and planes of closest fit to systems of points in space. *Philosophical Magazine 2*(11), 559–572.
3. Korte, A., & Farlow, A. (2013) The advantages and limitations of trait analysis with GWAS: a review. *Plant Methods* **9**, Article 29, https://doi.org/10.1186/1746-4811-9-29.
4. Flanagan, J. M. (2015). Epigenome-wide association studies (EWAS): past, present, and future. In M. Verma (Ed.), *Cancer Epigenetics*. Humana Press, pp. 51–63. https://doi.org/10.1007/978-1-4939-1804-1_3.
5. Wang, J., & Jia, H. (2016). Metagenome-wide association studies: fine-mining the microbiome. *Nature Reviews Microbiology* **14**, 508–522, https://doi.org/10.1038/nrmicro.2016.83.

6. John, O. P., & Srivastava, S. (1999). The Big-Five trait taxonomy: history, measurement, and theoretical perspectives. In L. A. Pervin & O. P. John (Eds.), *Handbook of Personality: Theory and Research* (Vol. 2). Guilford Press, pp. 102–138.
7. Curtin, P., et al. (2018). Dynamical features in fetal and postnatal zinc-copper metabolic cycles predict the emergence of autism spectrum disorder. *Science Advances* 4(5), eaat1293, doi:10.1126/sciadv.aat1293.

6

The Layers of Life

Emergent Complexity and Self-Organization

...and you may contribute a verse.

From *O Me! O Life!* by Walt Whitman

As we begin to conclude this book, we redraw the steps that led us here. We began this story by introducing the nature of time and of complexity, both in ourselves and in our environment, and in the interfaces between these complex systems that span many layers of organization. We traced the path that traditional structural perspectives have followed, always skirting the edges of time and complexity, from an initial rush of toxicological insights to the current deadlock that has paralyzed many parts of the field, adrift in an ocean of correlations. We sought to chart a new path forward, focused on the exploration of change at the interface of humans and their environment (Chapter 3) and the interdependencies that integrate us with our environment (Chapter 4) and through which we might redefine human health by the underlying patterns and forms that organize and constrain our biology (Chapter 5). But part of the challenge in defining a new perspective is in outlining the context from which this perspective emerges. Where does Environmental Biodynamics exist in relation to other important theoretical and methodological paradigms of today?

This is a critical issue for us because how this emerging field connects to the work of others is essential to its application in improving our health and our environment. We have argued in favor of shifting the fundamental framework

Environmental Biodynamics. Manish Arora and Paul Curtin with Austen Curtin, Christine Austin, and Alessandro Giuliani, Oxford University Press. © Oxford University Press 2022. DOI: 10.1093/oso/9780197582947.003.0006

of our studies away from a structural view alone to instead also embrace the dynamic complexity of our developmental biology. It is, therefore, apt to place our work within the framework of fields such as systems theory, which are attuned to dealing with constantly moving systems. By doing this, environmental health researchers, and epidemiologists especially, can find several important concepts already well developed and indeed flourishing, which will simultaneously allow them to leverage a wealth of theoretical knowhow while also extending the relevance of their own studies to new audiences.

General Systems Theory as a Unifying Framework

The emergence of general systems theory, a loosely defined interdisciplinary perspective, is often credited to the work of Ludwig von Bertalanffy, whose early efforts to create dynamical mathematical models of biological growth, and reconcile these with the laws of thermodynamics, became one basis for the general study of spatial and temporal systems.[1,2] This perspective was further advanced by mathematicians, biologists, psychologists, ecologists, and physicists to study a diversity of systems stretching from economics to biology to meteorology. Two prominent subfields to emerge from these pursuits, systems biology[3] and systems ecology,[4] are particularly relevant to the application of Environmental Biodynamics.

The most fundamental concept of general systems theory is unsurprisingly the notion of the *system*, a seemingly obvious amalgamation that ought to be simply defined in objective terms. This proves frustratingly difficult for biological and ecological systems because so few aspects of a given system, however defined, can be considered truly independent. How, then, does one define and dissect the organism from the environment, as each affect the other in a profound and vital ways, or the constituent components of each, as the functions of all are interdependent to some extent? Rather than being hindrances, from the view of general systems theory, it is these very interdependencies that provide the essential means of defining a system; that is, an organized entity consisting of interrelated and interdependent parts. The extent of interdependencies is naturally perspective-driven and thus, to some degree, subjective, but two natural boundaries for systems and their constituent components are in spatial and temporal organization. *A system is thereby defined as components that are structurally and/or functionally interdependent.*[5]

Many scientific approaches have been applied in studying complex systems, and we refer the reader to other publications for in-depth information.[6] We provide a figure that we have adopted from the work of Hiroki

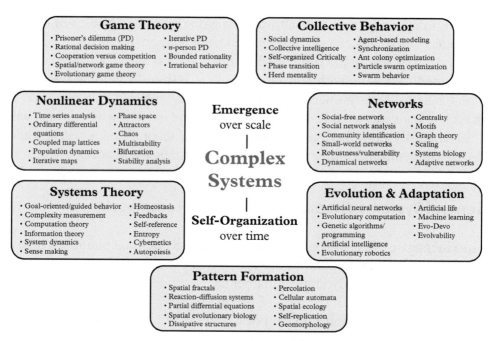

Game Theory
- Prisoner's dilemma (PD)
- Rational decision making
- Cooperation versus competition
- Spatial/network game theory
- Evolutionary game theory
- Iterative PD
- *n*-person PD
- Bounded rationality
- Irrational behavior

Collective Behavior
- Social dynamics
- Collective intelligence
- Self-organized Critically
- Phase transition
- Herd mentality
- Agent-based modeling
- Synchronization
- Ant colony optimization
- Particle swarm optimization
- Swarm behavior

Nonlinear Dynamics
- Time series analysis
- Ordinary differential equations
- Coupled map lattices
- Population dynamics
- Iterative maps
- Phase space
- Attractors
- Chaos
- Multistability
- Bifurcation
- Stability analysis

Emergence over scale

|

Complex Systems

|

Self-Organization over time

Networks
- Social-free network
- Social network analysis
- Community identification
- Small-world networks
- Robustness/vulnerability
- Dynamical networks
- Centrality
- Motifs
- Graph theory
- Scaling
- Systems biology
- Adaptive networks

Systems Theory
- Goal-oriented/guided behavior
- Complexity measurement
- Computation theory
- Information theory
- System dynamics
- Sense making
- Homeostasis
- Feedbacks
- Self-reference
- Entropy
- Cybernetics
- Autopoiesis

Evolution & Adaptation
- Artificial neural networks
- Evolutionary computation
- Genetic algorithms/programming
- Artificial intelligence
- Evolutionary robotics
- Artificial life
- Machine learning
- Evo-Devo
- Evolvability

Pattern Formation
- Spatial fractals
- Reaction-diffusion systems
- Partial differntial equations
- Spatial evolutionary biology
- Dissipative structures
- Percolation
- Cellular automata
- Spatial ecology
- Self-replication
- Geomorphology

Figure 6.1 An outline of general systems theory, based on the work of Hiroki Sayama.

Sayama (Figure 6.1) to summarize the various scientific disciplines pursuing the study of complex systems. Essentially, the purpose of general systems theory, whether applied in biological, ecological, social, or technological contexts, is in understanding interdependencies within and among systems. These include homeostatic mechanisms and adaptive responses, positive and negative feedback loops, and reciprocal interactions among system components and external environmental processes. These processes are discussed in more depth in Chapter 4. Here, we focus on two concepts that place Environmental Biodynamics within the unifying framework of general systems theory—*emergent complexity* and *self-organization*. These concepts are loosely defined in the literature and are at times used interchangeably; the nomenclature we use is intended only to provide a useful distinction between two general ideas that certainly intermingle, frequently overlap, and oftentimes collide.[7]

Emergent Complexity and Self-Organization

We will define emergent complexity as *some capacity or functionality in a system that is not apparent in the properties of its constituent parts*; it is the process by which new properties in a system develop as the scale and complexity of a system change. Emergence is a ubiquitous process that can be observed in any complex physical, biological, or social system that integrates multiple levels of organization. Consider, for example, the properties of hydrogen and oxygen, which as isolated elements are gases, and exhibit distinct characteristics and reactive properties. When these combine to form water, the resulting compound exhibits chemical and physical properties that neither constituent element is capable of—the fractal complexity of snowflakes, for example. In other words, we could analyze hydrogen and oxygen in their ionic form all we want, but we would not be able to fully predict the characteristics of the snowflake those elements are going to form.

Emergent complexity is ubiquitous in biological and ecological systems, as the processes mediating interactions at the molecular, cellular, and organismal levels of organization impose various interdependencies among themselves and give rise to new levels of organization.[8,9] This is true even at the level of whole animals and social systems; an ant is capable of a variety of tasks related to navigating and interacting with its world, but the ant colony, as a whole, processes information and responds to its environment with faculties beyond the scope of any given individual.[10]

Consider another example that is closer to human physiology and environmental exposures. At the simplest level of organization we are made up of atoms; actually just a few of the elements in the periodic table are the building blocks for life. At the next level, one with greater complexity, we see pathways that regulate proteins, fat, carbohydrates, and other molecules. Though these pathways comprise components derived from the first level, their mechanistic interactions at this level yield new biological functions; proteins interact with one another in ways that individual atoms cannot. At another level, where mechanisms and pathways derived from lower levels are integrated to form cells and circuits, we start seeing physiological dynamics emerge. These mechanisms are again composed of processes derived from lower levels, but their integration at this level yields new functional properties that were not apparent at the lower levels.

The novel functional dynamics that emerge across varying levels of complexity are also accompanied by changes in temporal dynamics. Consider that the interaction of synaptic processes will drive neurons to fire at scales spanning milliseconds to seconds; and, at the other end of the temporal spectrum, we have seasonal changes in our physiology where our biodynamics span several months. As these cycles determine not only our biological physiology but, at the highest level of organization, also our behavior, we see the emergence of ecological-scale rhythms. This takes us back to examples we mentioned in earlier chapters where our social behavior generates rhythms in air pollution emission and also drives our exposure to that very air pollution. At each of the levels in this example, there is a seeming paradox that is central to the concept of emergent complexity: Higher levels are composed of and are dependent on lower-level structures and functions *but cannot themselves be explained by the properties of the lower level.* For example, studying the atomic constituents of a human body does not allow us to accurately predict aspects of social behavior; rather, we would find informative data both at higher levels of organization within the individual and at different levels of organization in the environment (social and cultural norms, for example).

While emergence describes the appearance of new forms of functionality at higher levels of complexity, a related concept, self-organization, is essential to understanding how complexity emerges and propagates. *Self-organization* describes the patterns of organization that govern interdependencies among and between levels—the "rules" constraining the interactions at a given level. At the lowest levels of organization, for example, the availability of free energy and the stability of varying atomic species motivates chemical/ionic bonding that might catalyze the organization of complex molecules or drive molecular decay. As certain ions interact, reaching a level of molecular complexity, a new set of rules, driven by positive and negative feedback loops, propels the formation of more complex pathways. And, as these pathways interact, even more complex rules emerge, integrating multiple pathways and dynamic processes involved in cellular homeostasis. Emergence and self-organization are not limited to physical phenomenon, such as the formation of snowflakes, but are seen routinely in biological systems. In Figure 6.2 we show one example of this from bacterial cultures grown in a laboratory.[11]

The study of complexity thus involves characterizing not only the emergence of new biological functions at successive stages of organization but also the pattern of self-organization by which these systems organize, propagate, and maintain themselves. Through this lens, the focus of Environmental

(a)   (b)

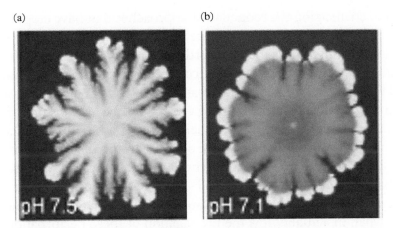

Figure 6.2 Emergence and self-organization of colonies of *Bacillus subtilis*. The pattern that the colony adopts is an emergent property—it is not available to any one individual bacterium but arises from the interaction of all the members of the colony. Furthermore, a shift in an environmental factor (here the pH) results in the change of the overall colony pattern, but different "rules" of self-organization drive the emergence of a different pattern.

Source: Tasaki S, Nakayama M, Shoji W (2017) Self-organization of bacterial communities against environmental pH variation: Controlled chemotactic motility arranges cell population structures in biofilms. PLoS ONE 12(3): e0173195. https://doi.org/10.1371/journal.pone.0173195.

Biodynamics, which we have emphasized in the context of a functional analysis of dynamic interfaces, is also an exploration of self-organization and emergent complexity.

Emergence and Self-Organization in Environmental Medicine

The relevance of emergent complexity and self-organization to environmental health research is twofold. First, given that the environment provides inputs to the body at all levels of organization—chemical, physiological, behavioral, social—and the body likewise impacts the environment on multiple levels, it is critical that we understand how interactions between our environment and our physiology propagate across different organizational tiers. Resolving this challenge will require examining how lower-level processes impact the emergence of higher faculties as well as understanding the self-organization of systems at each stage of organization. Second, these concepts are vital to challenging the reductionist approaches that have crept into environmental medicine. Case in point, we have seen at so many environmental epidemiology conferences that the word "mechanism," when used to provide biological plausibility to epidemiological findings, refers to some static, anatomical feature that exists at a more basic level of organization, most often a gene, an epigenetic mark, a protein, or a molecule. We have even heard claims that for every environmental input there must be a unique chemical signature in blood. This is wrong. In stark contrast to the theories of emergence and self-organization, such beliefs in environmental medicine research falsely imply that levels at smaller spatial scales are privileged in explaining causality (see the works of Denis Noble and Laurent Nottale that we have mentioned earlier), when in actuality it is the propagation of these perturbations across multiple levels of organization that leads to systemic dysfunction.

With the rise of -omic technologies, which can measure thousands of chemical signatures in biological and environmental samples, this issue has actually become more problematic because now we have an increased likelihood of finding false correlations between environmental factors and our physiology. We can avoid the confusion generated by the ocean of correlations implicit to high-dimensional data analysis by embracing a sound theoretical framework, which at its core must focus on the perturbation of self-organization and propagation of emergent complexity to produce a tangible gain in our understanding of human physiology. As we are writing this book, a very nice opinion piece has been published in a leading scientific journal. Paul Smaldino from the University of California very eloquently argues that in the world of ever-increasing scientific data, sound theories are more important than ever. Better theories will lead to better hypotheses, which will give rise to better models and methods to collect data, and all of this will operate in a "virtuous cycle."[12]

While the theoretical and methodological approaches we are discussing are uncommon in environmental medicine, in other fields they are making strong headway. Consider, as examples, these three studies at very different levels of organization that embraced a systems theory approach to study complexity. Tsuchiya and colleagues, for example, analyzed expression of mRNA in embryonic stem cells to identify mechanisms involved in cell differentiation.[13] Using data from the whole genome, they reconstructed attractor potential energy landscapes, similar to what we have previously shown in the metabolism of essential elements, to characterize the emergence of stable states and identify critical transitions between states. The formation of stable attractor states and the transitions between them are the "rules" we discussed previously in characterizing self-organization—the interdependent processes through which a system arrives at a stable dynamic at a given level. Such an approach could be leveraged to connect measures of self-organization at the transcriptomic level, as Tsuchiya and colleagues did, to link these processes to later stages of complexity, such as the health of an organ, system, or whole person.

At the larger scale of microbes, Lahti and colleagues studied emergent complexity and self-organization in the human microbiome, characterizing differential attractor landscapes organizing internal microbial populations (the "gut microbiome") at different timepoints in the human lifespan.[14] Similarly, and yet again at another ecological scale entirely, here involving the dynamics organizing whole ecosystems, Hirota and colleagues identified attractors underlying critical transitions between tropical forests and savanna grasslands.[15] From these studies, we can see that by focusing inquiry on global measures of organization and complexity, a system can be characterized in terms of organizational complexity and emergent dynamics, independent of the scale of the system itself, as these studies did from the level of the transcriptome and microbiome to ecosystems bigger than major cities.

What is the lesson here for environmental health researchers? It is that there are universal laws at play that operate at all physical scales, and we should leverage these phenomena to better understand how the environment and human physiology influence each other. However, the additional challenge facing us in health sciences is that we need to understand not only how complex systems emerge and self-organize but also what causes them to break down and spiral toward disease.

How Does Environmental Biodynamics Fit into Systems Theory?

The answer to that question is this: *Dynamic interfaces are necessary for emergence and self-organization of human–environment interactions.*

By learning from the works of many great scientists we have mentioned throughout this book, we have argued that one of the reasons we are unable to predict the emergence of complex behavior from one level to the next—for example, how studying atoms of hydrogen and oxygen cannot shed light on the final form of the snowflake—is because we are again assuming that the interactions between the systems at each level of complexity involve a direct transfer of information. In doing so we are ignoring the *operational independence* of dynamic interfaces and the fact that the interfaces mediate and constrain the transmission of information between levels. We have demonstrated that, at least in some aspects of health, the dynamics that emerge at the level of chemical–environmental interfaces allow the prediction of complex emergent phenomena, such as social affect–related dysregulation in autism.

Throughout this book we have argued that whether we are concerned with organization over space or time, we are dealing with change, and that change has a shape and the interfaces, or more precisely the processes that make up the interfaces, operate at different spatial and temporal scales so that the "shape of change" is constrained (or guided) by underlying rules that operate in space and time. The other contribution to the phenomena of emergence and self-organization comes from the dynamic interdependence axiom of our theory, which posits the interdependence and the fundamentally *embedded* nature of dynamic interfaces, which argue against them operating in isolation. All of these aspects of Environmental Biodynamics (and the biodynamic interface theory, which is at the core of this field) are necessary for emergence and self-organization.

In the most forthright terms, we argue that by including a thorough and direct analysis of dynamic interfaces, we do not have to just accept emergence and self-organization as universal phenomena; rather, we can actually begin to explain them. This is a bold claim, and we accept that much work is still needed to fully realize this claim. As we have done throughout this book, we want to back our claim with the data we have collected. For this, we will return to our work on autism spectrum disorder and direct your attention to Figure 6.3. From the level of individual ions where we measured zinc and copper orbits to the level of metabolic networks of the joint interaction of various essential nutrients and toxic chemicals, and from there to the next-higher levels of organization and scale where we studied the functioning of the brain and of whole individuals, we have seen how dynamic interfaces played an important role in deciphering interactions between our physiology and our environment. In Figure 6.3 we summarize that work by depicting different levels of organization included in our studies, but as you review the different levels shown in the figure, ask yourself this: *What lies in the seemingly empty space that connects the vastly different levels that operate at different temporal scales shown in the figure?*

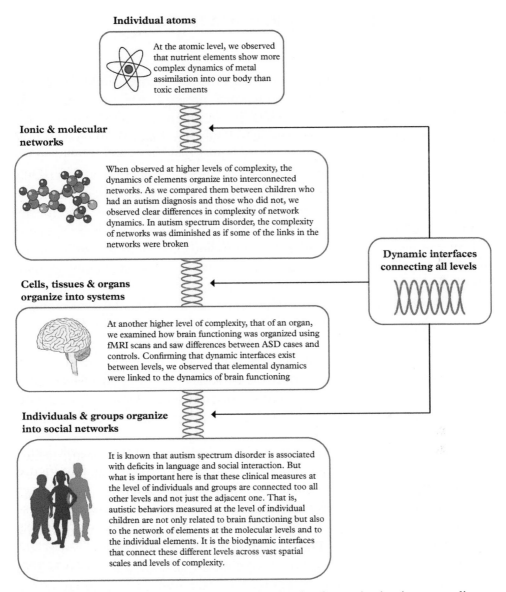

Individual atoms

At the atomic level, we observed that nutrient elements show more complex dynamics of metal assimilation into our body than toxic elements

Ionic & molecular networks

When observed at higher levels of complexity, the dynamics of elements organize into interconnected networks. As we compared them between children who had an autism diagnosis and those who did not, we observed clear differences in complexity of network dynamics. In autism spectrum disorder, the complexity of networks was diminished as if some of the links in the networks were broken

Dynamic interfaces connecting all levels

Cells, tissues & organs organize into systems

At another higher level of complexity, that of an organ, we examined how brain functioning was organized using fMRI scans and saw differences between ASD cases and controls. Confirming that dynamic interfaces exist between levels, we observed that elemental dynamics were linked to the dynamics of brain functioning

Individuals & groups organize into social networks

It is known that autism spectrum disorder is associated with deficits in language and social interaction. But what is important here is that these clinical measures at the level of individuals and groups are connected too all other levels and not just the adjacent one. That is, autistic behaviors measured at the level of individual children are not only related to brain functioning but also to the network of elements at the molecular levels and to the individual elements. It is the biodynamic interfaces that connect these different levels across vast spatial scales and levels of complexity.

Figure 6.3 Biodynamic interfaces connecting levels of organization in our studies on autism spectrum disorder.

How Does This Perspective Relate to Traditional Structural Views?

While emphasizing the separation between Environmental Biodynamics and traditional structural perspectives, it is worth noting as well that both seek to address a common set of questions relating the environment to human health; the differences between these views lie in how each evaluates the role of time and the nature of complexity. Both perspectives seek ultimately to explain the origins of health, which we will consider as a form of phenotype; a typically healthy person might be considered one phenotype, while the emergence of disease might be considered another. The structural perspective views the determination of a healthy or unhealthy phenotype as the interaction of genetic and environmental factors—the endogenous and exogenous determinants we introduced in Chapter 2. We could thus reconstruct this philosophy in algorithmic terms as $P = G \times E$, where P is the spectrum of health phenotypes and $G \times E$ reflects the interaction of genetic and environmental determinants. The underlying principle of $G \times E$ is that the health risk imparted by a set of genetic factors is modified by environmental factors, and, vice versa, that the health risk of environmental exposures is mediated by one's genetically determined constitution. In other words, a person is born (or conceived) with a genetic code that increases their predisposition to a healthy or diseased state, and the phenotypic expression of this genotype depends on their exposure to a set of environmental factors.

Contrary to historical perspectives on genetic determinism, which envisioned the genome as the direct determinant of ultimate phenotype fate (i.e., $P = G$), this perspective recognizes the role of the environment as a mediator of genetic pathways to phenotypic traits, a modifier of genetic traits via epigenetic mechanisms, and itself an initiator and driver of phenotype being modified by genetic input. There is nonetheless a critical flaw in the $G \times E$ formulation, even within the context of a purely structural framework: This formulation completely ignores the role of *time*, when in fact we know that the developmental age of an environmental exposure is critical to the role of that exposure in a person's development. One might therefore be tempted to modify the structural formulation to account for this, as: $P = \dfrac{G \times E}{T}$, where the newly included term T reflects the developmental timing (or age) of the genomic and environmental interaction, thereby capturing the notion of *critical windows of development* that is central to the concept of the Developmental Origins of Health and Disease (DoHAD).

Our modification of the traditional structuralist perspective may reconcile this view to current advances in developmental biology, but how could a functional view be represented in such a context? We suggest a new framework to capture this:

$$P = G \times E \times \frac{\Delta(G \times E)}{T}$$

This formulation emphasizes two critical insights advanced by Environmental Biodynamics. As articulated in prior models, the key elements in the determination of phenotype (P) are interaction of the genotypic (G) and environmental determinants (E), but here these elements are modified by a derivative term, $(\Delta(G \times E))/T$, which captures the incremental change (Δ) in gene–environmental factors over time. This explicitly captures the critical concept in Environmental Biodynamics, which emphasizes the significance of *time* in resolving biological mechanisms. From this perspective, the importance of genetic and environmental determinants cannot be assessed in the context of static measures but rather must include the variance of these measures over time. In contrast to the notion of time as a stratifying device, as in $P = (G \times E)/T$, where $G \times E$ reflects static measures whose significance may vary over time, here $G \times E$ factors are inherently time-varying and functional because their significance is modified by past as well as present values. In that sense, the periodic, recurrent, and functional nature of $G \times E$ factors is as critical a determinant of phenotype as are the structural properties of $G \times E$.

Implications of Environmental Biodynamics for Environmental Health Sciences

If, as proposed here, the effects of environmental inputs on human physiology are mediated by dynamic interfaces that have to date been unexplored, then their characterization can only propel us toward a better understanding of environmental health. We hope to enculture this new field of inquiry to shift the current focus from efforts to measure more and more exposures at lower and lower concentrations to identifying dynamic processes that assimilate exposures into human physiology. It will also require a shift from trying to identify which exposures impact human health to identifying how the process of environmental exposure impacts human health; that is, rather than examining purely structural aspects of exposure, we should be considering the underlying patterns in the temporal organization of exposure metabolism.

To realize the full potential of Environmental Biodynamics, environmental medicine must refocus the examination of the interaction of environment and health from an emphasis on measuring physiological "moments" (i.e., static measures of environmental factors, infrequent anthropometry, momentary health indicators) to studying dynamic human–environment interfaces, physiological states, and the processes that constrain those states. To this end, we provide a set of endeavors that must be undertaken to capitalize on and formally test the biodynamic interface paradigm:

1. **To focus our scientific inquiry on interfaces that connect biological and environmental systems.** An important consequence of the conjecture we propose is that studying the input and output systems will not permit complete characterization of the interface. The interface is not a derivative of either system; it must be studied directly. Given that the interface may exhibit complexity independent of the systems contributing to its emergence, we must focus on the characteristic emergent complexity, self-organization, state dependency, and sensitivity to initial conditions. In practice, this can be achieved by implementing the methods outlined in Chapter 3, focusing on the underlying attractor systems and related dynamics that govern biodynamics over time.

2. **To develop theoretical frameworks that focus on the identification and interpretation of *constraints* in biological–environmental interfaces.** The constraints acting upon a given interface will ultimately determine the organization of the interface, its response to perturbation, and subsequently the phenotypic "output" signal. Analyzing correlations between different measures of the environment and human physiology without characterizing the constraints will not yield a satisfactory explanatory model. To achieve this, environmental science should focus on the exploration of underlying patterns, forms, and networks connecting embedded systems.

3. **To develop laboratory, clinical, and epidemiological methods** to relate the complexity characterized at the level of biodynamic interfaces to human health, particularly with regard to the interfaces of processes that unite humans and their environments. We need to measure processes with better characterization of organizational levels *and time*. Explicitly,

this requires the rejection of epidemiological study designs that ignore processes and measure the environment and human physiology as static entities. At a conceptual level, we must reject a purely structural reductionist perspective. At an operational level, we suggest the adoption of mathematical methods already well established in other disciplines, particularly systems biology and statistical physics. These include methods appropriate for characterizing the phenomenological nature of a given system, and its dependency on varying inputs and underlying processes. For example, the application of Takens embedding theorem;[16,17] recurrence quantification analysis to measure signal periodicity, entropy, and determinism;[18] potential energy analysis to identify transitions in underlying attractors;[19] and the empirical estimation of Lyapunov exponents[20–22] to characterize stochastic, deterministic, and chaotic processes underlying a given system are well-characterized methods suitable to achieve these goals, which should be complemented by the development and application of newer approaches to data analysis.

Our Verse (Conclusion)

We are taught that an atom is made of electrons moving around a nucleus containing protons and neutrons. What is often overlooked is that one of the most important components of an atom is the seemingly empty space between the electrons and the nucleus. Without this space, matter as we know it would cease to exist. The importance of that space is not that it separates the atom's electrons from its nucleus, but that it is where so much happens—that space is where electrons interact with the nucleus of their own atom. When an atom is perturbed (by the ingress of energy in the form of X-rays during fluorescence, for example), it is this space where electrons rearrange themselves to achieve a stable configuration. It is also this seemingly empty space where electrons from one atom interact with those of other atoms, and thus chemical reactions, including those that gave rise to life, begin. The same is true when we look upwards to the heavens—between all the planets, moons, comets, and stars that are out there, there is that essential emptiness, the space that facilitates gravity, radiation, and the evolution of our physical universe.

Why should it be any different in the medical sciences? Throughout this book, we have highlighted the works of others that reject homeostasis in favor of homeodynamics,[23] that extend relativistic concepts from physics to

---

Box 6.1 Poetic Aside

Clay is molded to make a pot,
but it is in the space where there is nothing
that the usefulness of the clay pot lies.

Therefore, benefit may be derived from something,
but it is in nothing that we find usefulness.

excerpt from Lao Tzu, *Tao Te Ching*,
translated by Victor H. Mair

---

biology,[24] that accept the developmental stages of our biology and argue for the existence of critical windows of susceptibility,[25] and that study human biology as a network of systems. Many of these scientific theories and methods rely on the existence of levels, scales, and states defined by their properties, and compartments defined by their structures and/or functions. Because of this, the direction of causality across levels and scales has been, and rightly so, the focus of much scientific debate. These levels, scales, and compartments are necessary, but let us not forget that equally necessary is what exists between them. In this book, we have turned our gaze to this seemingly empty and undefined space, and in doing so, we have presented an argument not about the direction of causality between systems and their components, but where causality exists, and what makes causal linkages possible—*dynamic interfaces*.

References

1. von Bertalanffy, L. (1968). *General Systems Theory: Foundations, Development, Applications*. George Braziller.
2. Hammond, D. (2019). The legacy of Ludwig von Bertalanffy and its relevance for our time. *Systems Research and Behavioral Science* **36**(3), 301–307.
3. Kitano, H. (2002). Systems biology: a brief overview. *Science* **295**(5560), 1662–1664.
4. Odum, H.T. (1983). *Systems Ecology: An Introduction*. Wiley.
5. Montuori, A. (2011). Systems approach. In M. Runco & S. Pritzker (Eds.), *Encyclopedia of Creativity* (2nd ed.). Academic Press, pp. 414–421. doi:10.1016/B978-0-12-375038-9.00212-0.

6. von Bertalanaffy, L. (2015). *General Systems Theory: Foundations, Development, Applications*. George Braziller.

7. Halley, J., & Winkler, D. (2008). Classification of emergence and its relation to self-organization. *Complexity* **13**(5), 10–15.

8. Coffey, D. S. (1998). Self-organization, complexity and chaos: the new biology for medicine. *Nature Medicine* **4**, 882–885, doi:10.1038/nm0898-882.

9. Benci, V., & Freguglia, P. (2004). About emergent properties and complexity in biological theories. *Rivista di Biologia* **97**, 255–268.

10. Millonas, M. M. (1992). A connectionist type model of self-organized foraging and emergent behavior in ant swarms. *Journal of Theoretical Biology* **159**(4), 529–552, https://doi.org/10.1016/S0022-5193(05)80697-6.

11. Tasaki, S., Nakayama, M., & Shoji, W. (2017). Self-organization of bacterial communities against environmental pH variation: controlled chemotactic motility arranges cell population structures in biofilms. *PLoS One* **12**, e0173195, doi:10.1371/journal.pone.0173195.

12. Smaldino, P. (2019). Better methods can't make up for mediocre theory. *Nature* **575**, 9, doi:10.1038/d41586-019-03350-5.

13. Tsuchiya, M., Giuliani, A., Hashimoto, M., Erenpreisa, J., & Yoshikawa, K. (2016). Self-organizing global gene expression regulated through criticality: mechanism of the cell-fate change. *PLoS One* **11**, e0167912, doi:10.1371/journal.pone.0167912.

14. Lahti, L., Salojarvi, J., Salonen, A., Scheffer, M., & de Vos, W. M. (2014). Tipping elements in the human intestinal ecosystem. *Nature Communications* **5**, 4344, doi:10.1038/ncomms5344.

15. Hirota, M., Holmgren, M., Van Nes, E. H., & Scheffer, M. (2011). Global resilience of tropical forest and savanna to critical transitions. *Science* **334**, 232–235, doi:10.1126/science.1210657.

16. Takens, F. (1981). Detecting strange attractors in turbulence. In D. Rand & L-S. Young (Eds.), *Dynamical Systems and Turbulence, Lecture Notes in Mathematics* (Vol. 898). Springer-Verlag, pp. 366–381.

17. Abarbanel, H. (1996). *Analysis of Observed Chaotic Data*. Springer-Verlag.

18. Marwan, N., Romano, M. C., Thiel, M., & Kurths, J. (2007). Recurrence plots for the analysis of complex systems. *Physics Reports* **438**, 237–329, doi:10.1016/j.physrep.2006.11.001.

19. Livina, V. N., Kwasniok, F., & Lenton, T. M. (2010). Potential analysis reveals changing number of climate states during the last 60 kyr. *Climate of the Past* **6**, 77–82, doi:10.5194/cp-6-77-2010.

20. Bryant, P., Brown, R., & Abarbanel, H. D. I. (1990). Lyapunov exponents from observed time-series. *Physical Review Letters* **65**, 1523–1526, doi:10.1103/PhysRevLett.65.1523.

21. Kim, B. J., & Choe, G. H. (2010). High precision numerical estimation of the largest Lyapunov exponent. *Communications in Nonlinear Science and Numerical Simulation* **15**, 1378–1384, doi:10.1016/j.cnsns.2009.05.064.

22. Takens, F. (2010). Reconstruction theory and nonlinear time series analysis. In H. W. Broer, B. Hasselblatt, & F. Takens (Eds.), Handbook of Dynamical Systems (vol. 3). Elsevier, pp. 345–377.

23. Lloyd, D., Aon, M. A., & Cortassa, S. (2001). Why homeodynamics, not homeostasis? *ScientificWorldJournal* 1, 133–145, doi:10.1100/tsw.2001.20.

24. Noble, D. (2012). A theory of biological relativity: no privileged level of causation. *Interface Focus* 2, 55–64, doi:10.1098/rsfs.2011.0067.

25. Wright, R. O. (2017). Environment, susceptibility windows, development, and child health. *Current Opinion in Pediatrics* 29, 211–217, doi:10.1097/MOP.0000000000000465.

Appendix
Operationalizing Environmental Biodynamics

One way to define or measure the value of an idea is by the solutions or new approaches it offers. Simply put, this sounds something like "if we think things work like *this*, then we should do *that*." The ideas offered in this book suggest new ways to think about connections between individuals and their environment; we question the existence of hard boundaries between these systems and focus instead on the interfaces that emerge between them, which derive from the properties of each. In this appendix, we focus on the implications and applications of these ideas; that is, what we should *do* with Environmental Biodynamics.

We approach this topic through the lens of three essential components of operationalizing a scientific theory into a scientific study: (1) the questions one must ask, (2) the measures one should take, and (3) the means to analyze and interpret these outcomes. As well, we consider the practical and theoretical implications of these approaches, which will have ramifications for environmental health study design. While this approach is intended as a broad guide to the application of Environmental Biodynamics, we anticipate that both the technological and mathematical examples we cite will become outdated; that is a good thing to happen because thriving scientific fields advance rapidly but don't forget their origins. And as much as these ideas may guide study design and fieldwork, we suggest as well that these provide an ideal introduction for students and teachers interested in incorporating Environmental Biodynamics into their studies.

The Questions Defining an Environmental Biodynamics Approach

At the heart of any scientific study are the fundamental questions it seeks to answer. These questions may emerge inductively from the need to explain a series of observations or they may be deduced from a prior theoretical model, to evaluate their extension to a new case. The question is usually couched in the formal language of a hypothesis, which allows for its falsification and, as well, embeds the question in an empirical context.

In environmental health sciences, questions typically take a general form similar to "Does exposure to a toxic chemical during early life lead to adverse neurodevelopmental outcomes?" And the hypothesis that follows grounds this in both an empirical and a falsifiable context: "Greater exposure to that toxic chemical will be associated with worse performance on an intelligence test." The study design that emerges from this fundamental question would lead one to measure chemical biomarkers in early life (pregnancy, at birth, or in infancy, for example) and test at a later age if performance on IQ tests was worse in kids who experienced more exposure to the chemical of interest at those times. This is a perfectly reasonable approach, but, as discussed in Chapter 2, the implicit assumption underlying questions such as these is that the fundamental connection between developing children and their environment is driven by *structural* dependencies; that is, the type of chemicals they are exposed to, and the amount of the exposure.

Environmental Biodynamics seeks to evaluate *functional* dependencies between environmental and biological systems, and as such requires a different set of fundamental questions and hypotheses. Here, we suggest three general categories of inquiry around which to organize Environmental Biodynamics studies, and practical hypotheses that may be advanced in this framework to study the role of functional dependencies in how our environment impacts our health.

Set 1: On the Organization of Systems

Question 1: What Is the Nature of Complexity in This System?

The first and most fundamental questions considered in an Environmental Biodynamics approach relate back to the concepts introduced in Chapter 1, paraphrasing the scheme proposed by Warren Weaver. That is, we must ask three questions:

1. Is the system driven by simple, deterministic connections between a small set of elements ("organized simplicity")?
2. Does the system reflect the action of a multitude of probabilistic factors ("disorganized complexity")?
3. Or, instead, does the system involve the action of multiple, embedded, and hierarchical processes ("organized complexity")?

In practice, while it may be impossible to fully describe the interdependencies that organize a given system, we can define or distinguish between these by the manner in which the systems behave. If we may sufficiently describe a system through a simple, deterministic equation—Ohm's law, for example, where the current through a given circuit is proportional to the ratio of voltage and resistance—then a reasonable description of the system is that of organized simplicity. And, knowing this, we might approach our measurement and analysis of the system through the lens of those simple constituent processes. However, when the system we observe yields seemingly stochastic patterns of change—white noise, for example, where power is equally distributed among all frequencies, which are equally likely to occur—we might infer a system of disorganized complexity. And, last, we might characterize organized complexity in the emergence of hierarchical patterns and interdependencies—when the effect of Variable A is dependent on the activation of

Process B, which is mediated by Process C, and Processes B and C are linked by positive and negative feedback loops that mediate their intermittent activation over time.

Addressing these questions does not necessarily provide the answer to a given study in itself; rather, it informs the researcher how a given system *should* be studied. Systems that can be explained through simple deterministic interactions can reliably be profiled with linear, differential, and related deterministic equations; likewise, stochastic systems are best explained through the lens of probabilistic mechanics. This is in fact the most common framework in which systems involved in environmental health are currently investigated. In the prior example of chemical exposure and cognitive development, for example, the measures of both the toxic chemical and IQ are presumed to occur more or less at random, and we test, on average, how the distribution is shifted with varying chemical exposure. Complex systems, on the other hand, may require more sophisticated assessments involving the simultaneous measurement of multiple processes in order to unravel the dependencies among them. Importantly, an adequate study of complex systems must consider temporal dynamics of the interacting systems and the biodynamic interface that emerges from that interaction; it is through this lens, and in the dynamics of the underlying attractor system, that the "rules" that organize a given system become apparent.

As we have discussed in this book, the nature of complexity in a given system should be the necessary first step in any investigation, but for a variety of reasons most published environmental health studies have proceeded with little consideration of this point; for a given environmental factor of interest, studies might focus on whether the linkage between input and output reflects a simple determinism, a noisy association, or the superimposition of inputs on ongoing processes such as persistent metabolic dynamics. If, like us, environmental scientists see the folly in ignoring the nature of complexity, Environmental Biodynamics presents all of with us a new frontier full of opportunity.

Question 2: How Is Complexity Organized in This System?

Distinguishing between simple, disorganized, and complex systems provides an essential basis for determining how a given system should be studied, but the researcher still must decide how to measure and define the system at hand. In the practice of environmental epidemiology, using essentially observational study practices, we hardly ever know the literal equations governing a given system we are beginning to study. However, we still have tools that can point us in the right direction—for example, we can use *attractor reconstruction*, as outlined in Chapter 3. The attractor, reflecting the set of points toward which a given system converges, describes a map of all possible states in a given system. By reconstructing the attractor underlying a given system, we can identify the patterns around which it is organized and distinguish, for example, the orbits of a periodic or chaotic system from the central tendencies of a stochastic system. Beyond providing the direction of further inquiry, the attractor in itself provides a basis for measuring the dynamics governing a given system. We have outlined several methods for achieving this, particularly recurrence and cross-recurrence quantification analysis, but there are also a wide array of methods that might similarly be applied to this end, for example the estimation of Lyapunov exponents, cross-convergent mapping, and related methods based on attractor reconstruction, as explained later. In this manner, the organization of complexity leads naturally to a context of hypothesis testing. For example, if one were applying recurrence quantification analysis to analyze determinism in the metabolism of a toxic chemical, one might ask whether a more deterministic metabolism of that chemical in early life relates to later-life childhood IQ. Likewise, to extend beyond a simple probabilistic framework and consider the emergence of organized complexity, one might use similar dynamical metrics to construct network-based analyses, structural equation modeling, and latent factor methods.

Question 3: At What Temporal and Spatial Scales Does Complexity Emerge?

A subtle but essential question underlies the aims and feasibility of the preceding inquiries; that is, at what scale do I measure complexity? Recall the example of a hypothesized pendulum from Chapter 2, which at one sampling resolution appears as a persistent light, at another resolution as a persistent absence of light, and, finally, at an appropriate resolution, as an oscillating pendulum. In proposing that we define the nature of complexity in Question 1, and in describing its organization with attractor reconstruction in Question 2, we have taken for granted that the researcher has characterized the system at an appropriate spatial and temporal scale in order to capture the essential variability that will describe the system at hand. How, in practice, does the research determine the appropriate scale? There are no easy answers to this question— we cannot, for example, always use the finest resolution that can be practically achieved because this can be misleading, as was the case in the hypothesized pendulum example where Lab 4 picked the finest resolution but all sampled within a narrow time window. Another way to conceptualize this issue is to think in terms of looking down the eyepiece of a light microscope—we keep adjusting the focus until we can see the object of interest clearly. We purposely overshoot and then return to the clearest view to make sure we are at the best focal length. For environmental epidemiology, the "appropriate" scale is essentially the temporal resolution that allows one to address Questions 1 and 2—that is, the scale that allows one to characterize the dynamics in the system. We gave an example of this in Chapter 2 where we discussed that to capture the true dynamic nature of the pendulum system, we would have to vary the temporal resolution of our measurements and observe the systems at different sampling resolutions—this is similar to the light microscopist varying the focal length at which they observe the object of interest. Ultimately, a temporal scale that yields insufficient samples to characterize a pattern of change is by definition inadequate to characterize functional dynamics. Note the enormous implications this holds for traditional study designs that focus on assessing environmental inputs from a single biomarker or infrequently measured biomarkers—from this perspective, much of the past 50 years of progress in studying the health impacts of environmental inputs has been built on an inappropriate scale. The potential opportunities for new discoveries in linking functional complexity in these systems to health outcomes are endless.

Set 2: On Constraints and Interdependence

Question 4: What Patterns Drive and Constrain Complexity in a Given System?

In Chapter 5 we discussed the simple example of the spatial dimensions (length, width, thickness) of a turtle's shell, and how variability in one dimension ultimately determines another. In simple terms, a shell that is long will also be wide, for example; the length of the shell constrains the width, and vice versa. Likewise, in considering complexity in the interfaces between individuals and their environment, we must seek the patterns and constraints that determine how that complexity will emerge. A diet high in one essential element may likewise be high in others, for example. These constraints might be identified through the lens of dimensionality reduction techniques such as principal component analysis, or through the investigation of multiple agents through the use of mixtures models, which seek to identify combined or aggregate effects rather than consider effects in isolation. In the context of hypothesis testing, one might relate dynamics measured in the principal components of a given system to a given health outcome; for example, *Does greater determinism in this underlying metabolic factor relate to higher performance on an IQ test?* Again, the central idea here is that the nature of hypothesis testing does not shift with the embrace of a functional analysis; rather, the process one measures and relates to an outcome has changed.

Question 5: How Is complexity in One System Embedded in Others?

This topic, which we approached throughout the book but in most detail in Chapter 4, is particularly pernicious in biological systems driven by *organized complexity*. For the researcher, these systems can be particularly difficult to characterize adequately, as they require time-resolved measurements of multiple processes. We have been able to achieve this in studying environmental chemical inputs, particularly essential and toxic elements, by using lasers to map the growth rings in teeth to generate detailed temporal profiles of environmental exposures. We emphasize that these are by no means the only methods one might use to characterize environmental health dynamics and highlight several comparable approaches later in this chapter. We want to emphasize to students of environmental health sciences that, while the challenges are great in capturing so-called deep data, so are the opportunities. It is our contention that it is not only entirely plausible, but also the norm, that the complexity driving a given individual's health is driven by the integration of multiple complex systems—and that it is only possible to fully characterize this complexity through the exploration of time-varying dynamics. To leverage this, researchers can embrace high-dimensional analyses of system dynamics, particularly network analyses and graph theory–related measures, which provide new metrics to describe a system. In this context, hypothesis testing follows in relating health outcomes with measures derived from network and graph theory, such as clustering coefficients, centrality, between-ness, and so forth.

Set 3: On Emergence and Self-Organization

Question 6: Ultimately, How Does the Organization of Complexity in Biodynamic Interfaces Drive Human Health?

The business of answering Questions 1 through 5 will involve the measurement of a given environmental input in an individual (for example, a biomarker of uptake of environmental exposures), the reconstruction and measurement of an attractor system that includes aspects of the input and the physiological system's response (thus, the interface), and the derivation of parameters that characterize and quantify complexity at the level of the interface. The point of all this hard work is to yield measurements of complexity that can ultimately be related to human health and development in meaningful ways. Throughout the book, we have outlined a number of examples relating measures derived from recurrence analysis of elemental metabolism to several different disease states, including autism spectrum disorder and other neurological conditions. Notably, these studies included explicit traditional hypothesis tests (e.g., whether higher determinism in elemental metabolism relates to the risk of being diagnosed with autism spectrum disorder) as well as predictive contexts (e.g., whether we can predict disease from metabolic dynamics). These approaches can pave the way for a truly personalized environmental science grounded in explanatory and predictive functional analyses.

Empirical Methods to Study the Organization of Environmental Biodynamics

While Environmental Biodynamics may offer new questions to ask, to achieve our goals there must also be a shift in the empirical methods we use to achieve them. Given that Environmental Biodynamics focuses on resolving the temporal organization of complex systems, it should be clear that the primary requirements for these studies are temporally resolved data. This is somewhat in contrast to the dominant paradigm currently emerging in the fields of environmental health sciences at present, which is focused on the extension of -omics approaches. Following advances in genomic sciences, which seek to characterize the complete human genetic sequence, environmental health scientists likewise seek to characterize the totality of environmental exposures that may manifest in biomarkers in human tissue. The mapping of the human "exposome" is a vast endeavor made possible by recent advances in mass spectrometry, particularly so-called untargeted mass spectrometry, which may simultaneously sample many tens of thousands, and inevitably hundreds of thousands, of chemicals in a single tissue sample. Environmental health science has, in other words, advanced to the age of Big Data science.

But for Environmental Biodynamics, the utility of these advances is questionable. There is of course an obvious, compelling need and attraction in measuring more and more things. But, so long as these measures are taken as static measurements assessed at a given timepoint, we must question the capacity of this approach to truly capture the complexity underlying a system. How, for example, could one characterize interdependencies between environmental and biological systems (positive and negative feedback loops, rhythms, regime shifts, and many others) with information derived from a single timepoint or a few timepoints? If one recalls the hypothesized example of a pendulum light studied at multiple temporal resolutions, we would essentially be making the same mistake made in those approaches but replicated many thousands of times over.

To address these shortcomings and to develop a more functional scientific perspective, Environmental Biodynamics proposes that the future of environmental health sciences lays in a *Deep* Data approach. In contrast to current Big Data -omic approaches, which capture many measures simultaneously at a single timepoint or a few timepoints, the Deep Data approach describes the *successive* measurement of a given system over time. This approach is the essential foundation to any Environmental Biodynamics study, as it is in the temporal dynamics of a given system that the organization of complexity becomes apparent. In practice this can be achieved from two perspectives we briefly outline here, which focus on either the *retrospective* reconstruction of prior exposures or the *prospective* collection of ongoing exposures.

Biological Hard Drives and Retrospective Exposure Reconstruction

Here, we consider characteristics of biomatrices that would allow the retrospective assessment of exposure timing without repeated collection of biological samples. We consider these characteristics analogous to those of electronic hard drives that capture and archive digital information in a manner that preserves the sequential order during the input of information for faithful retrieval at a later timepoint.

The ideal biomarker must be a faithful archive not only of the intensity or dose of exposure but also of the *timing* of exposure. For temporal exposure information to be faithfully recorded, the biological matrix used for exposure assessment must have an incremental structure that allows delineation of exposures at different timepoints. To achieve this, a matrix must accrue the environmental chemical (or its metabolite) in an incremental fashion with exposure from different time periods being captured in discrete compartments that can be analyzed separately. We provided the example of assays performed on human teeth to uncover exposure timing, which has been the focus of our work, but similar attributes may be extended to other matrices such as hair and bones. The incremental nature of teeth may be visualized as "growth rings" where each ring/increment carries distinct temporal information and is chronologically related to the adjacent rings, thereby forming a sequential increment of information. Of course, not all studies will have access to teeth, so we provide a general framework that can be used when considering the attributes of biomatrices that can provide temporal information on environmental inputs and physiological responses.

Archival and Stable

While many tissues in the body develop incrementally, few provide a stable archive of information that is not corrupted over time and may be decoded retrospectively to obtain the timing and intensity of past exposure. The major reasons behind the loss of the original imprint of exposure are tissue remodeling and exchange (both uptake and outflow) with circulating fluids. This impacts not only commonly used biomatrices such as blood or urine that show relatively regular turnover for many chemicals but also tissues such as bones that undergo periodic remodeling during growth spurts or periods of bone resorption.

Multiple Exposures

Ideally, the biological matrix being assayed captures exposure information for multiple classes of environmental inputs. In the case of chemical exposures and their metabolites, it is also important that the chemicals that are captured in the biomatrix and accumulate at levels that can be detected and quantified with current technology.

Accessible and Ethical

A biological matrix for assessing exposure must be readily sampled without the need for invasive procedures, which limit its use in epidemiological investigations. As examples, we have noted the advantages of teeth over blood and urine; however, a major limitation of using tooth-based biomarkers is that they cannot be obtained, at least not ethically, prior to natural shedding, which happens after the age of five to six years for most children. By this age, many conditions, such as autism, are clinically detectable, and critical windows for prevention or mitigation of severity have been missed. Blood and urine, on the other hand, can be ethically collected from birth, and umbilical cord blood provides a window into the prenatal environment at birth, which are significant advantages over teeth and other media that are only accessible much later in life. The ethics of biomarker selection and their analysis are also points of consideration. For example, umbilical cord blood is only available at one time and once used cannot be replenished. Use of assays that are not state of the art, then, calls into question the appropriate use of a finite resource.

Biomonitoring and Prospective Exposure Sampling

With retrospective exposure reconstruction methods one seeks to dive into the past and characterize what has happened; at the same time, current and future technological advances will make it possible to monitor the present in sufficient resolution that we might have advance warning of an adverse future trajectory. Examples of similar approaches currently abound in the marketplace, particularly in the area of wearable fitness devices that persistently measure daily steps, activity, heart rate, temperature, and other physiological indicators. Much like the example analyses of weight loss and cardiac rhythm we presented in Chapter 3, prospective physiological data collection at an appropriate temporal sampling resolution can be used to map interfaces between our physiology and our behavioral environment.

At the time of the writing of this book, prospective exposure sampling at the level of the individual remains somewhat in its infancy. Although wearable devices exist to monitor exposure to certain environmental inputs and, in fact, are necessary tools in certain occupations, these typically lack the sensitivity and specificity of more traditional laboratory assessments, are prohibitively expensive, and/or may be too complex for convenient and persistent use.

Even in the present state of development, persistent physiological monitoring opens avenues and opportunities for interface-based analyses. For example, data on heart rate collected by wearable fitness monitors might be used for attractor reconstruction and thereby characterize the cardiac interface; paired with traditional "static" -omic assessments, it would at least be possible to link structural determinants at the environmental level to interface dynamics at the physiological level. As such, prospective monitoring devices may present important opportunities for advancing Environmental Biodynamics and hold tremendous potential for the future.

Computational Methods to Study the Organization of Environmental Biodynamics

The general focus of computational methods grounded in a traditional structural perspective is to characterize the distribution of cross-sectional measurements, and to identify factors relevant to this distribution. One might think of this as how a measure, for example height, is organized in a population and what factors relate to this organization. Were you to measure height in some population, or a likewise similarly continuous measure, you might find a bell-shaped Gaussian distribution, such that the greatest frequency (most common height) clusters around the mean. We might extend this perspective to an inferential framework by testing if, for example, the mean height differs between males and females. In a simple, practical sense the computational language one falls into thus involves either a linear association between continuous measurements, or the comparison of central tendencies between groups, for example, or testing if the distribution of some exposure variable in a given population relates to the odds of an individual being in one group or another. These forms of hypothesis testing can all be implemented through some generalization of the general linear model (e.g., ANOVA, correlation, and logistic regression).

These frameworks are equally useful in the practical application of Environmental Biodynamics, with the essential caveat that a preliminary step is needed to derive appropriate metrics characterizing functional dynamics in retrospective or prospective signals. With these data, measures relevant to a population distribution hold little relevance at the level of the individual, both because each measurement is not independently sampled and because a central tendency tells us little about a dynamic or trend over time (although other measures, such as variance and deviation, might). Instead, the essential primary goal is to derive measurements that describe the pattern of underlying dynamics in a system. Typically, this begins through the lens of attractor reconstruction, which in the context of Environmental Biodynamics, where the measurement reflects time-varying inputs to a biological system, is the fundamental unit of the biodynamic interface.

Here we outline a variety of computational methods that might be applied to retrospective or prospective environmental health data, as outlined in the prior section. We emphasize that this brief survey is intended only to provide examples intended to point readers in some useful directions; this is by no means an exhaustive review. We also emphasize that these topics are ongoing areas of method development and innovation, and so it is entirely possible that novel methods and approaches will be available that may supersede these approaches. That said, the general approaches we outline share a common theme in that each is approached through a broad lens and is outlined toward the specific goal of addressing research questions in Environmental Biodynamics, as introduced earlier in this chapter.

Lagged Embedding and Attractor Reconstruction

In Chapter 3 we introduced the notions of attractor reconstruction and lag embedding following the method introduced by Floris Takens, now known as the Takens theorem.[2] This approach is used to reconstruct the underlying attractor governing a given series of sequential measurements, and as such plays an essential role in Environmental Biodynamics. At the level of a qualitative analysis, attractor reconstruction can be used to distinguish between stochastic and periodic systems by the formation (or absence) of periodic behaviors, which manifest in constrained orbital trajectories. Purely stochastic systems, in contrast, yield an "attractor" organized only in relation to some central tendency, with no time-varying influence of one moment upon another. As such, attractor reconstruction is the first step toward addressing Question 1 (posed earlier in this chapter) as it provides a simple basis for characterizing the organization of a given system. As well, and as expanded upon later in this appendix, attractor reconstruction is usually an essential first step in the application of subsequent analyses that can be used to derive quantitative metrics of system dynamics.

Determinism, Periodicity, and Entropy: Recurrence Quantification Analysis

While attractor reconstruction is used to reveal the underlying processes governing a system, this does not in itself necessarily yield the quantitative metrics one might wish to *measure* in a system. Recurrence quantification analysis (RQA)[3–5] and multivariate extensions of RQA, particularly cross-recurrence quantification analysis (CRQA), are a family of descriptive analytical methods that can be used to quantify periodic and state-dependent dynamics in an attractor. The general focus of the method involves the application of a threshold function to each point in an attractor in order to define a system *state*; then, the temporal intervals between recurrences to a state are measured and used to construct a recurrence plot, from which one can derive a series of computational metrics. Metrics we have found particularly useful in characterizing biodynamic interfaces in exposure metabolism include (1) determinism, which measures the prevalence of periodic processes in an attractor system; (2) entropy, or rather Shannon entropy, a metric derived from information theory that describes the complexity of a given measure; and (3) diagonal length, which measures the mean duration of periodic processes.

Relating to the questions posed earlier in this chapter, particularly Questions 2 and 6—that is, how complexity is organized, and how this organization relates to health—RQA and related metrics can be used to operationalize Environmental Biodynamics in a practical hypothesis-testing framework. For example, given a retrospective or prospective measurement of environmental inputs, one might apply RQA to measure *determinism* and test if, for example, this feature relates to a given health outcome. In Chapter 3 we discussed a study in which we applied this method in a similar framework to identify dysregulated metabolism of essential nutrients in autism spectrum disorder.

Potential Energy Landscapes and Regime Shifts

Potential energy analysis[6] is another tool useful in the exploration of attractor dynamics, particularly in the exploration of bistable systems, bifurcations, and other indicators of the underlying self-organization of a given system. Like RQA and related methods, this approach relies on the evaluation of a time series; however, rather than characterizing the evolution of a system through a reconstructed phase space, potential analysis focuses on identifying the propensity for *change* associated with varying levels of systemic activity. The logic underlying this approach is that a system, while operating by the dynamics of an attractor, will tend not to diverge from the variability associated with an attractor state; as such, if we observe an abrupt shift in system variability, then this may reflect a shift from one attractor to another. Such shifts are common in bistable systems, as outlined in the circuit introduced in the introduction to Chapter 4; that is, a system that is alternatively governed by one attractor or another. As such, potential analysis provides a useful tool for understanding the self-organization of complexity in a given system (i.e., the "rules" that it follows). Scientists have applied this approach to achieve better understandings of systems spanning multiple levels of organization, from climate dynamics[7,8] to microbiology,[9] ecological transitions,[10,11] and metabolic dynamics.[12]

Potential energy analysis allows us to identify the peaks in potential energy, which reflect unstable transition points between systems, and the valleys that likewise indicate the formation of stable states, where, for a time, a system is likely to remain in a given state. We have introduced applications of this approach at two levels of organization. The first is in characterizing the formation of bistable systems in elemental metabolism, and the dysregulation of these processes in amyotrophic lateral sclerosis. Likewise, at a second stage of organization, we have extended this approach to the analysis of neuroimaging data, as shown in Chapter 4, in order to characterize shifts in persistent states in neural activity. In a similar vein, future studies can leverage potential analysis and related methods to investigate the organization of environmental health; that is, how the "rules" that govern elemental metabolism persist or shift over time, and how the maintenance or breakdown of these processes relates to human health. In parallel to the application of attractor reconstruction and RQA/CRQA, this provides an approach to addressing Questions 1 and 2—that is, measuring the organization and complexity of a given system—and in relating these measures to human health, as per Question 6.

Cross-Convergent Mapping, Dynamic Connections, and Temporal Interdependencies

The methods summarized so far have focused on the analysis of either a single retrospective or prospective signal, or, in the case of CRQA, the extension of univariate methods to a bivariate case. There is an equally important need, particularly in addressing Questions 4 and 5, to understand how the dynamics in a given system relate to, constrain, or depend on the dynamics in related systems. To achieve this, we here highlight cross-convergent mapping (CCM),[13-15] a method that, much like RQA, begins with an initial focus on attractor reconstruction. Rather than focusing explicitly on periodic and state-dependent dynamics, CCM seeks to characterize the extent to which dynamics in one attractor are driven by another and to identify the temporal separation in these processes—that is, if change in one attractor manifests in another contemporaneously or if there is a lag between change in one system and an effect in another. In our studies, we have applied CCM to characterize how attractor dynamics involved in the metabolism of essential elements drive one another, and to characterize the lag involved in this process. Findings from our preliminary investigations suggest that both the intensity of connections between elements and the lag between cause and effect are indicative of disease.

While the explicit focus on attractor reconstruction lends itself to the theoretical basis of Environmental Biodynamics, CCM is by no means the only potential approach to characterizing dynamic temporal dependencies. A diverse array of related methods might similarly be applied toward the same goal. In particular, the estimation of Granger causality, a related dynamical metric that similarly seeks to characterize the link between variability in one system and another, may be particularly fruitful to Environmental Biodynamics studies, as it has been widely applied in related fields such as structural neuroimaging.

Dimensionality Reduction and Network Construction

It should be evident that the application of any of these descriptive analyses to retrospective or prospective data will yield a broad array of functional measures. For example, if one were to generate a retrospective analysis of, say, five environmental inputs to a given individual and then apply RQA/CRQA, potential energy analysis, and CCM to every possible permutation of dependencies between and among systems, then one might be left with many dozens of measures, each providing a different metric characterizing complexity within and among systems. In that sense dynamical measures can sometimes present a sort of dimensional expansion in that a single time series can become dozens of measurements, each describing a different aspect of how the system is organized. How can we make sense of such high-dimensional complexity?

In Chapter 5 we addressed this question from several angles, particularly focusing on the general principles of dimensionality reduction. In brief, this involves the derivation of a lower-dimensional space—that is, some set of latent factors or components, in essence a new (smaller) set of measurements—that can represent the variability observed across the full array of measured variables. This sort of approach has a number of advantages both theoretically and in practice. From a conceptual standpoint, the focus on the underlying dimensions, factors, or components driving the overall system can provide a more interpretable summation of a given system, while simultaneously allowing the specification of what constraints, correlations, and co-dependencies relate each variable to another. And, in practice, the components/factors derived through these methods can reduce the need for multiple hypothesis tests and thereby bolster statistical power.

In Chapter 5 we also provided an example illustrating the construction of a network—in our context, a metabolic network—derived from the application of RQA to multiple environmental inputs (essential elements primarily derived through diet). Much like attractor reconstruction, the construction of a network allows a global perspective on the organization of a given system and likewise provides the basis for subsequent quantitative analysis. Graph theory, in particular, is useful in the analysis of networks, providing a quantitative means to characterize how central any given feature is to a network, how many other features it is connected to, and the relative complexity of direct and indirect pathways between that feature and others.[16,17] In practice, the application of this approach might therefore involve characterizing, as an example, how recurrence dynamics for a given environmental input relate to dynamics in other inputs and comparing, relatively, how different elements are more or less dependent on others. Likewise, as metabolic networks are characterized in healthy individuals, this approach can be extended to characterize the dysregulation of metabolic networks in disease. In sum, when applied in a functional context, this approach allows direct measures of the constraints and dependencies that drive the emergence of dynamics in different systems, and can thereby be an important tool in addressing Questions 4 and 5.

Design and Theoretical Implications

We began this appendix by considering what can be achieved with Environmental Biodynamics. We proposed, as a first step, the consideration of a new set of questions relating to the topics explored in Chapters 1 through 6; these would direct the research to consider the nature of complexity in a given system, to characterize it and relate it to other systems, and ultimately to link these processes to human health. We next outlined the need for retrospective and prospective empirical methods that would yield Deep Data sufficient to explore complexity in environmental exposures and metabolism. Last, we outlined some computational approaches relevant to these tasks. Here, we consider the implications of these approaches to theoretical models and ongoing study design.

It seems appropriate that initial applications of Environmental Biodynamics should focus on the validity and utility of this theoretical perspective itself. As the goal of any theory is to describe, explain, predict, and manipulate the world, it seems only appropriate that Environmental Biodynamics should be evaluated by its efficacy in those contexts. To that end, we have described a number of studies demonstrating the utility of the Environmental Biodynamics framework in (1) characterizing complexity in elemental metabolism; (2) relating this to explanatory models that identify dysregulation in autism and related developmental disorders as well as amyotrophic lateral sclerosis; and, likewise, (3) constructing predictive models useful in forecasting disease. These studies demonstrate the usefulness of Environmental Biodynamics across multiple populations, life stages, and disease states.

By the same token, these initial applications of Environmental Biodynamics are exactly that: a series of initial studies. Future work must continue to demonstrate the efficacy of this approach if it is to provide a useful complement or alternative to the dominant structural paradigm. Particularly critical to this process will be extending biodynamics beyond the evaluation of essential and nonessential elements, which were the basis for most of the work described to date. We must discover, in other words, if the patterns we observe are general principles of human physiology or discrete patterns that emerge in elemental metabolism. As well, future studies must extend this work beyond the disease areas we outline, which, while including markedly different disorders, commonly focus on neurological impairment.

From the perspective of epidemiological study design, the nature of hypothesis testing in an Environmental Biodynamics framework is largely unchanged; instead, it is the focus of measurement that has shifted. For future researchers this creates the heavy burden of shifting their empirical methods to the generation of Deep Data through prospective or retrospective sampling methods and the corresponding adoption of computational methods to appropriately characterize these data. But even with those changes the essential nature of hypothesis testing remains the same: Rather than test if the magnitude of an exposure relates to a health outcome, Environmental Biodynamics will test if complexity involved in exposure metabolism relates to the outcome instead. This common hypothesis-testing framework thus provides the means by which the ongoing validation and evaluation of Environmental Biodynamics may continue; that is, its usefulness as a theory will ultimately depend on the utility of the hypotheses it generates. Ultimately, what one should *do* with Environmental Biodynamics is go out and practice it. This will mean measuring environmental inputs to biological systems, describing the patterns these inputs form over time, and relating those patterns to the health of the biological system.

References

1. Weaver, W. (1948). Science and complexity. *American Scientist* **36**(4), 536–544.
2. Takens, F. (1981). Detecting strange attractors in turbulence. In D. Rand & L.-S. Young (Eds.), *Dynamical Systems and Turbulence, Lecture Notes in Mathematics* (Vol. 898). Springer-Verlag, pp. 366–381.

3. Eckmann, J., Oliffson, S., & Ruelle, D. (1987). Recurrence plots of dynamical systems. *Europhysics Letters* **5**, 973–977, doi:10.1209/0295-5075/4/9/004.

4. Marwan, N., Romano, M. C., Thiel, M., & Kurths, J. (2007). Recurrence plots for the analysis of complex systems. *Physics Reports* **438**, 237, doi:10.1016/j.physrep.2006.11.001.

5. Marwan, N. (2008). A historical review of recurrence plots. *European Physical Journal Special Topics* **164**, 3–12, doi:10.1140/epjst/e2008-00829-1.

6. Nolting, B. C., & Abbott, K. C. (2016). Balls, cups, and quasi-potentials: quantifying stability in stochastic systems. *Ecology* **97**, 850–864, doi:10.1890/15-1047.1.

7. Livina, V., Kwasniok, F., Lohmann, G., Kantelhardt, J. W., & Lenton, T. M. (2011). Changing climate states and stability: from Pliocene to present. *Climate Dynamics* **34**, 2437–2453.

8. Livina, V., Kwasniok, F., & Lenton, T. M. (2010). Potential analysis reveals changing number of climate states during the last 60 kyr. *Climate of the Past* **6**, 77–82.

9. Lahti, L., Salojarvi, J., Salonen, A., Scheffer, M., & de Vos, W. M. (2014). Tipping elements in the human intestinal ecosystem. *Nature Communications* **5**, 4344, doi:10.1038/ncomms5344.

10. Dakos, V., et al. (2012). Methods for detecting early warnings of critical transitions in time series illustrated using simulated ecological data. *PLoS One* **7**, e41010, doi:10.1371/journal.pone.0041010.

11. Hirota, M., Holmgren, M., Van Nes, E. H., & Scheffer, M. (2011). Global resilience of tropical forest and savanna to critical transitions. *Science* **334**, 232–235, doi:10.1126/science.1210657.

12. Curtin, P., et al. (2020). Dysregulated biodynamics in metabolic attractor systems precede the emergence of amyotrophic lateral sclerosis. *PLoS Computational Biology* **16**, e1007773, doi:10.1371/journal.pcbi.1007773.

13. McCracken, J. M., & Weigel, R. S. (2014). Convergent cross-mapping and pairwise asymmetric inference. *Physical Review E: Statistical, Nonlinear, and Soft Matter Physics* **90**, 062903, doi:10.1103/PhysRevE.90.062903.

14. Schiecke, K., Pester, B., Feucht, M., Leistritz, L., & Witte, H. (2015). Convergent cross mapping: basic concept, influence of estimation parameters and practical application. *Proceedings of the Annual International Conference of the IEEE Engineering in Medicine and Biology Society* **2015**, 7418–7421, doi:10.1109/EMBC.2015.7320106.

15. Ye, H., Deyle, E. R., Gilarranz, L. J., & Sugihara, G. (2015). Distinguishing time-delayed causal interactions using convergent cross mapping. *Scientific Reports* **5**, 14750, doi:10.1038/srep14750.

16. Gross, T., & Sayama, H. (Eds.). (2009). *Adaptive Networks: Theory, Models, and Applications*. Springer-Verlag.

17. Guzzi, P., & Roy, S. (2020). *Biological Network Analysis: Trends, Approaches, Graph Theory, and Algorithms*. Academic Press.

Index

For the benefit of digital users, indexed terms that span two pages (e.g., 52–53) may, on occasion, appear on only one of those pages.

Figures and boxes are indicated by *f* and *b* following the page number.